NOT OUR KIND OF GIRL

NOT
OUR KIND
OF GIRL

Unraveling the Myths
of Black Teenage Motherhood

ELAINE BELL KAPLAN

WITH A FOREWORD BY
ARLIE RUSSELL HOCHSCHILD

UNIVERSITY OF CALIFORNIA PRESS
BERKELEY   LOS ANGELES   LONDON

University of California Press
Berkeley and Los Angeles, California

University of California Press, Ltd.
London, England

©1997 by
The Regents of the University of California

Library of Congress Cataloging-in-Publication Data
Kaplan, Elaine Bell.
    Not our kind of girl : unraveling the myths of black teenage
    motherhood / Elaine Bell Kaplan : with a foreword by Arlie
    Russell Hochschild.
        p. cm.
    Includes bibliographical references and index.
    ISBN 0-520-08736-4 (cloth: alk.paper). — ISBN 0-520-
20858-7 (pbk. : alk. paper)
    1. Afro-American teenage mothers—Case studies. 2.
Teenage Pregnancy—United States—Case studies. I. Title.
HQ759.4.K36 1997
306.874'3—dc21   96-46709
                                                    CIP

Printed in the United States of America
9 8 7 6 5 4 3 2 1

To Lewis and Daveed

When you're in a hostile environment that doesn't tell you what you can really expect from that environment, and it just goes on and on, it's something that becomes a part of you. And you don't know any better or know any different.

Evie Jenkins, teen mother

Contents

Contents

Foreword: An Inner City
of the Heart

In the 1950s, 25 percent of all Black households with children in America were headed by single mothers; by 1990 the number had increased to 61 percent. Of these single-parent families, more than half have daughters who themselves are or will become teen mothers. Some scholars implicitly challenge the assumption that teen pregnancy is really a "problem," arguing that, statistically, a poor Black woman is no more likely to get a good job or a good husband if she has a baby at twenty-five than if she has one at fifteen. But Elaine Bell Kaplan sees teen pregnancy as a symptom of a very deep problem we have barely begun to understand.

In *Not Our Kind of Girl* Kaplan cuts through the simplifying stereotypes of both conservative and liberal explanations—that the teen mother has "bad values" or is a "helpless victim"—by exploring the complex context and the feelings of the teenager herself. In the tradition of Lillian Rubin's *Worlds of Pain,* Kaplan conducts us through the jarring world of the teen mother. She takes us up ill-lit, narrow staircases into the cramped apartments of public housing projects. We sit with her on a bench amidst broken glass in a drug dealers' park. We follow her into militarized high school classrooms and the offices of overworked, worried counselors. We go with her as she helps a teen mother move from one apartment to another—one of the invisible transients, as some call them. With keen insight and empathy, Kaplan describes the unmet needs of developing daughters, the rageful disappointment of struggling mothers, the fear that their boyfriend will disappear. Drawing from her study of thirty-two teen mothers and adult women who were once teen mothers, Kaplan reveals a rich variety of patterns with a common thread: many girls she comes to know are living in an emotional inner city.

Kaplan takes a hard look at current theories for why teens become mothers. For some, Black teen mothers live in a self-perpetuating "culture of poverty" that can be turned around only by adopting the values of marriage and hard work. But the girls she studies, Kaplan counters, already want a loving husband, a good job, and a nice house. Often their mothers even more earnestly want these things for them. They *have* family values.

For more economically oriented thinkers, such as William Julius Wilson, Black teen mothers are indirect victims of deindustrialization. The flight of jobs from inner cities, Wilson argues, robs Black men of blue-collar employment that enables them to become reliable providers and caring fathers. In the absence of marriageable men, women have children on their own.

Still other studies, such as Carol Stack's *All Our Kin,* suggest that the Black kin system functions as a mutual aid society by helping to raise the children of single mothers. But Kaplan discovers a threadbare, overstretched kin system and shows that, poverty aside, inner-city Black mothers lack the informal social ties that support middle-class women, both Black and White.

It is the absence of support, Kaplan argues—especially from parents—that best explains why teenagers get pregnant and decide to keep their babies. Just at a point in life when young girls need affirmation, many feel unloved by their mothers, ignored by their schools, and rejected by their fathers and boyfriends. The girls' mothers are anxious, distracted, often in poor health, and worn down by the struggle to raise a family in a virtual war zone. Understanding their mothers' weariness but unable to turn elsewhere for familial affection, they continue to want and need mothering. Surrounded by people, they feel isolated. A baby represents a way of making a relationship—by making someone to have a relationship with. They are "relationship-poor." In having a baby, they hope to become "relationship-rich."

Kaplan dismantles a number of myths about the families of teen mothers. Many people believe that inner-city Black parents condone their daughters' pregnancies. Kaplan shows, on the contrary, how desperately mothers want their daughters to finish high school, marry, and prepare for a good job. They scold their daughters, often beg them to end the pregnancy, sometimes banish them from the house. The pregnancy almost always precipitates a crisis in the family and aggravates already strained relations. As one girl Kaplan calls Evie says, "My mother hated me for it. I was just alone. . . . She just couldn't stand to look at me. I had to go stay on my own for a while."

Kaplan explodes another stereotype as well. Some middle-class commentators assume that Black teenage girls enjoy a free and easy sexual life. We adults, Kaplan suggests, are perceiving Black teenagers "through our own steamy glasses." She finds that sex is a minimal part of the drama, rarely something the girls enjoy. Indeed, she reports, 60 percent of pregnant Black teenagers, according to one study, have been sexually abused as children. Pregnancy is perhaps a way of de-sexualizing themselves to avoid unwanted sexual attention.

Kaplan also insightfully describes the dilemma faced by the troubled mothers of pregnant teens. Some had themselves become pregnant "too early" and had struggled to overcome the attendant disadvantages. Wanting more than anything to see their daughters follow a different path, they experience their daughter's pregnancy as "one more cross to bear," a blow to their dreams and their motherly pride. Whether a mother supports her daughter, appearing to condone the pregnancy, or denies support, friends and neighbors may see her as a bad parent. In the eyes of the world, there is no way to appear a good mother; even in her own eyes, the road is unclear.

This important book helps us address a giant paradox posed by Andrew Billingsley in *Climbing Jacob's Ladder.* How can it be that a people who survived the brutality of slavery, endured the hostility of Reconstruction, and hung on through the discrimination and disadvantages of the modern era now seem to be succumbing to forms of self-destruction, such as Black-on-Black violence, drug addiction, and teen pregnancy?

In every form of oppression, if it truly succeeds, the oppressed "do it to themselves." Kaplan provides a key to understanding just how this invisible oppression works. Living in an inner city today is not simply a matter of cramped living quarters, run-down schools, and absent fathers, but also of severely damaged relationships. Look, she says, at the estrangement between this mother and daughter here and the rift between that teacher and student there. Look at the frayed bond between the teen girl and the father of her child. It is the injury to these vital bonds, this hidden oppression, that is the secret troublemaker.

What, then, are the political implications of Kaplan's work? It follows from her analysis that William Julius Wilson's proposed economic Marshall Plan for the inner city is necessary—but also not enough. If Kaplan's analysis is correct, we need not simply better schools but also better relationships between mentors and students. We need more jobs for men but also fuller support for men who try to be good fathers. We need better housing but also more mother-teen workshops, youth outreach programs, and other programs not yet devised because we haven't been thinking about "relational poverty." *Not Our Kind of Girl* is a wise, thoughtful book that can open the way to social policies that work.

Arlie Russell Hochschild

Acknowledgments

This study would not have been possible without the participation of the teen mothers, their families, and other women who took me into their homes and their confidence, and whose experiences presented me with a constant theoretical and practical challenge. I would like to give special thanks to the women in my Berkeley study group, Karen Dresser, Jane Singh, and Carolyn Stewart, for their faith in this project. They created a supportive intellectual environment for discussing ideas and putting the "taken for granted" in a new light. I must also thank Lucy De Pertuis for her critical analysis, insight, comments on a draft, and stimulating conversation about teenage mothers and sociology. Many others indirectly contributed to this project, among them Gloria Bowles, Dorothy Brown, Mary Jo Lakeland, Jacquelyn Marie, Phyllis Palmer—all gently guiding me through various stages of the research. Thanks to bell hooks for leading the way by reading the draft of her book on feminist theory to my women of color study group, and to Alice Walker for serving as a role model. All of these women have stood up for women like the ones in this study, and I thank them for showing me how to do the same.

During the early stages of this research, my dissertation committee was most supportive. I want to give warm thanks to Arlie Russell Hochschild for her guidance and for the telephone calls to see if I'm "there" yet. I continue to learn from her brilliant insights and observations about women and the sociology of emotion. Such ideas are the backbone of this study. Troy Duster and others, especially Janice Tanagwa, at the Institute for the Study of Social Change in Berkeley, were always willing to offer advice and support. Barbara Christian's own work on Black women's issues and her belief in this project were tremendously important to me. Michael Wiseman, a former dissertation committee member, who wrote pages upon pages of comments, also contributed to my work. Although he doesn't know it, Bob Blauner's red question marks on a paper I wrote for his class led to the development of the chapter on Black fathers.

Financial support came from the Institute for the Study of Social Change. The U.C. Berkeley Department of Sociology's Graduate Student Fellowship Fund also made the early part of the project possible.

This project started a dissertation, but it has been completely revised and by now little resembles the original manuscript—many of my ideas didn't coalesce until after the completion of the dissertation. In fact, I have worked continuously on refining the ideas while trying to stay up to date on the political thinking and scholarship concerning Black teenage mothers. To that end, I thank San Jose State University faculty grant funds for support. I owe much to Sharon Elise, Eun Mee Kim, Bob Massey, Rivka Polatnick, Claire Reinelt, Lillian Rubin, Karen Sacks, Richie Sanders, and Pierrette Hondagneu-Sotelo for reading and critiquing earlier drafts. They were so committed to understanding the issues in this book that we often spent hours in debate and discussion. Michele Fine discussed with me her work on adolescent girls. Kristen Luker read an earlier draft, let me see her work, and encouraged me to push further. Frank Furstenberg Jr. shared with me research on Black teenage fathers. Thanks to Barry Glassner for his faith in my ability to finish this work. A hundred kisses to Gwyneth Kerr Erwin for coming into my life with her green inked suggestions and her perceptive questions forcing me to make my ideas clearer. I received a great deal of encouragement from Naomi Schneider at U.C. Press, as well as from the anonymous reviewers whose critical comments contributed to the final product.

Other friends and family members gave me space and encouragement. My own family reminds me that we have more to learn about the Black family. Lewis and Daveed Kaplan have had more of an impact on this book than I can say. Lewis's critical comments and observations are always on the mark. I benefit greatly from his generosity of spirit, deep compassion for people who live on the margins, and sociological eye. A special thanks to my son Daveed for letting me use the computer, accompanying me to interviews, and being patient throughout this whole process. The prospect of spending more time with him and Lewis when I am done spurred me to complete this book. The support of all these people helped me bring this book to its conclusion.

Introduction

"If we want to solve the problems of the Black community, we have to do something about illegitimate babies born to teenage mothers." The caller, who identified himself as Black, was responding to a radio talk show discussion about the social and economic problems of the Black community. According to this caller's view, Black teen mothers' children grow up in fatherless households with mothers who have few moral values and little control over their offspring. The boys join gangs; the girls stand a good chance of becoming teen mothers themselves. The caller's perspective captures the popular view of many Americans: that marital status and age-appropriate sexual behavior ensure the well-being of the family and the community.[1]

Sixteen-year-old De Vonya Smalls's circumstances demanded a deeper interpretation. "I was fourteen when I first started having sex. I don't think I got pregnant the first time, maybe the third time. I cut school and went to his house. I was really in love." De Vonya, a tall and dark-complexioned mother of a nine-month-old baby, wore her hair in long, cornrow braids pulled tightly away from her slender face and favored jeans and bulky sweaters. She made these statements as we sat around a wobbly table in her friend's dimly lit kitchen. Nearby, a faded plastic shade flapped in the open window. De Vonya's words came with conviction and feeling. Despite her plain looks and tendency to speak slowly and softly, De Vonya often offered keen insight into her situation.

De Vonya's family had its fair share of problems. Her parents were poor, and her brothers and sisters were unemployed. Though she was the youngest of six children, she was not considered special or treated like the "baby" of the family. It was hard for the large family to treat anyone special. As soon as De Vonya's sisters and brothers were old enough, they left home. De Vonya had not seen her eldest brother in years. Her youngest brother was serving a three-year prison sentence for selling drugs. Her three sisters, all mothers recently separated from their husbands, were on welfare. De Vonya's father, a hospital orderly, left the family so long ago that she could not remember when he lived with them. She was angry at him: "He barely talked to me about anything." But she kept in touch with him, anyway. Recently, after suffering two heart attacks, he had quit his job, and he was now living on a small monthly disability insurance check.

De Vonya's mother raised the six children by working as a housekeeper for "rich White folks" who lived in the Oakland hills. Three years ago the doctor diagnosed De Vonya's fifty-two-year-old mother as having extreme hypertension. "Now she can't work," De Vonya explained to me. De Vonya had her own medical problems. When I asked why she did not use birth control, she told me, "The doctor says I can't use birth control because I've had two breast operations." De Vonya and her mother lived on a monthly disability check until she became pregnant and had to apply for welfare. The tensions between the two that had always been there but had never been fully expressed erupted at full force when De Vonya became pregnant.

Two weeks before our interview, De Vonya had moved out of her mother's East Oakland apartment because they had fought over her decision to keep her baby: "She asked me whether I was going to keep it and who's the father and where I was going to stay. I told her yeah, I was going to stay here. And she said, 'How do you know I want you to stay here? I've already raised my kids!' I never did tell her about the baby's father."

De Vonya Smalls was trying to achieve the American Dream. In her version of the Dream, having a baby was an act of individualism and achievement. But why would she choose that course? Why could DeVonya, an intelligent teenager, say, "I got pregnant because when I thought about it, I thought that maybe I could have somebody to love me better because I can't love my mother and she doesn't love me. Maybe I'll feel loved by having my own child"?

Girls like De Vonya stand in direct contradiction to the American
notions of family values and how one achieves the American Dream.
According to mainstream ideology, men who through hard work have
moved up the career ladder and provide their families with decent
food on the dinner table, clothes on their backs, and an occasional
family vacation have achieved the American Dream. Women's
achievements are measured by their marriage and child rearing, done
in proper order and at an appropriate age. Teenage girls are expected
to replicate these values by refraining from sexual relations before
adulthood and marriage.

Certainly, such traditional ideas held sway over the Black community I knew. Two decades ago unmarried teenagers with babies
were a rare and unwelcome presence in my Harlem community.
These few girls would be subjected to gossip about their lack of
morals and stigmatized if they were on welfare. But by the 1980s
so many young Black girls were pushing strollers around inner-city
neighborhoods that they became an integral part of both the reality and the myth concerning the sexuality of Black underclass culture and Black family values.[2] These Black teenage mothers did
not fit in with the American ethic of hard work and strong moral
character.

As early as the 1800s, as Alexis de Tocqueville described, the American people believed that individuals are free to think, live, work, and
participate in any setting they choose.[3] Anyone, Americans tout, can
surmount racial, sexual, and class barriers in America if they have the
"right stuff." We often hear stories of people who have climbed out of
poverty, achieving wealth and glory through sheer grit and determi-
nation. Even those who are Black and poor believe the American
Dream is a great equalizer. Those who have not succeeded obviously
have not tried.

If this conservative ideology is extended to teen mothers, their situation can be explained only as a result of aberrant moral character. If
Black adolescent girls fail to achieve, something in their nature pre-
vents them from doing so. As president, Ronald Reagan often urged
teenage mothers to "just say no" so that taxpayers would no longer be
forced to pay for their sexual behavior. The "Just Say No" slogan in-
voked by the Reagan and Bush administrations in the 1980s was uti-

lized in the 1990s by both Black and White conservatives in the attempt "to change welfare as we know it."[4] If these politicians have their way, teenage mothers will be shunned, hidden, and ignored.

As I made my way through East Oakland and downtown Richmond to interview teen mothers,° I witnessed a different scenario from the one devised by politicians. Teenage mothers are housed in threatening, drug-infested environments, schooled in jail-like institutions, and obstructed from achieving the American Dream. In our ostensibly open society, teenage mothers are disqualified from full participation and are marked as deviant. Black teenage girls aged fourteen, fifteen, and sixteen—many of them just beginning to show an adolescent interest in wearing makeup, dressing in the latest fashions, and reading teen magazines—are stigmatized. These teen mothers attempt to cope as best they can by redefining their situation in terms that involve the least damage to their self-respect.

Are Black teenage mothers responsible for the socioeconomic problems besetting the Black community, as the radio show caller would have us believe? Do Black teenage mothers have different moral values than most Americans? Do they have babies in order to collect welfare, as politicians suggest? Do the families of Black teenage mothers condone their deviant behavior, as the popular view contends? Or, as William J. Wilson's economic theory suggests, is Black teenage motherhood simply a response to the economic problems of the Black community?[5] Black teenage girls confront a world in which gender norms, poverty, and racism are intertwined. Accordingly, to answer questions about these young mothers, we must sort out a host of complex economic and social problems that pervade their lives. I hope the questions I have asked and the answers given will provide portraits of real teenage mothers involved in real experiences.

The reality of these teenage mothers is that they have had to adopt strategies for survival that seem to them to make sense within their

---

°Except when necessary for clarification, all teenage mothers and older women who were previously teenage mothers will for the sake of brevity be referred to as teen mothers—a term they use. When appropriate the teen mothers' own mothers will be referred to as adult mothers. All names and places have been changed to protect confidentiality.

social environment but are as inadequate for them as they were for teenage mothers in the past. As I emphasize throughout this book, my observations of these teenage mothers' home lives do not reveal a deviant culture. Nor does the ethnography show that teenage motherhood is accidental. What stands out for me in De Vonya's comments at the beginning of this Introduction is the possibility that motherhood may be related not only to socioeconomic status but also to the psychological growth of adolescent girls.

This book is organized in three parts, as follows. In Part I, Chapter 1 outlines some of the theoretical perspectives social scientists use to explain Black teenage motherhood. This chapter also discusses social and economic changes that have effectively stripped Black families of their social support base. Chapters 2 and 3 describe the lives of the teen mothers who took part in the extensive portion of the study. Chapter 2 examines the assumption of sexual permissiveness among Black teenage mothers and shows how it contradicts the teenage mothers' actual attitudes. In Chapter 3 a few teen mothers talk about their daily lives, the problems they confronted before becoming pregnant, and why they became pregnant. Together these chapters depict the complexities of being a Black teenage girl. Part II describes what happens to families as social support systems when they become burdened by teenage motherhood. Chapters 4 through 6 explore the strain that teenage pregnancy and motherhood can cause in young mothers' intimate relationships. The notions of motherhood and fatherhood are examined, as well as the impact that parenthood has on the teenage mothers' decision making.

In Part III, Chapters 7 and 8, I follow the teenage mothers into the welfare office, community meetings, and peer group settings, where they must learn strategies to handle the stigma of being teenage mothers. This interaction with the community shows how it deals with members seen as reinforcing a so-called deviant image. Particularly in Chapter 9, and generally throughout this book, *Not Our Kind of Girl* demonstrates that we examine Black teenage mothers within larger social, historical, and ideological frameworks.

Finally, I will suggest that these ethnographic pictures illuminate the way structural contradictions act on psychological well-being and the way people construct and reconstruct their lives in order to cope on a daily basis. One issue that comes through quite clearly in this study, and one that is often overlooked by politicians and various studies on Black teenage mothers, is that these teenagers know what constitutes a successful life. Black teenage mothers in this book struggle against being considered morally deviant, underclass, and unworthy.

If we are to understand the stories of these teenage mothers and generalize from their experiences in any significant way, we must place them within the current theoretical and political discussions concerning Black teenage mothers. As T. S. Eliot noted long ago, reality is often more troubling than myth.

Part One

Myth versus Reality

Chapter One

Black Teenage Mothers

Becoming a Social Problem

My God, that should be a Cabbage Patch baby in that bassinet. I said, "Can you believe that's yours?" I told her, "You need to stop having sex."

Ann Getty, teen parent counselor

In Black America many teenage girls become mothers before they complete their education, even before they reach maturity. The rising number of girls with babies is evidence of the changing structure and dynamics of Black family life.[1] The number of Black households headed by single Black women with children climbed from a low of 25 percent in the 1950s to 61 percent by the early 1990s. Of these families, more than half have daughters who were or will become mothers during their teenage years.[2]

The birth rates among Black teenage girls aged seventeen and younger have climbed during the past forty years, making the Black birth rate for this age group two to three times that among White teenagers. In 1991 alone, over 150,000 of these teenagers under the age of twenty had given birth to children. Although the birth rate among Black teenage girls has declined somewhat in the past few years, it is still double that among White teenage girls. The majority of Black teenage mothers are poor, surviving on a low income or on welfare.[3]

3

The Culture-of-Poverty Perspective

Alarmed by the rising numbers of babies born to unmarried and poor teenage girls, scholars began to take note of what they saw as a serious social problem in the Black community. Oscar Lewis was the first social scientist to use the term *culture of poverty*, which later became synonymous with the social problems researchers saw in Black culture. According to Lewis, poor people who live in a capitalist industrial society have developed certain cultural characteristics, such as an absence of childhood and a high percentage of mother-centered homes. These characteristics have produced survival strategies enabling the poor to adapt to conditions of poverty but making it difficult for them to escape their situation. That is, poverty creates even more problems for poor communities and consequently causes poverty to be passed from one generation to the next.[4]

In 1965 Daniel Patrick Moynihan advanced the culture-of-poverty thesis in a report that had tremendous implications for Black teenage mothers. According to Moynihan's perspective, poor and segregated populations such as the Black community develop a distinctive set of beliefs, values, and behavior patterns perpetuating their condition. For instance, Moynihan notes that more Black than White families are headed by poor women. He interprets the increasing rates of mother-only Black families as a sign that the structure of the Black family is deteriorating. Black mother-only families appear unstable, producing uncontrollable children, the boys joining gangs and the girls becoming sexually active at an early age. Moynihan's perspective suggests that Black teenage girls' morals are different from those of mainstream society because they do not have strong moral values prohibiting sexual activity at an early age and before marriage.[5]

Missing from Moynihan's culture-of-poverty argument is any suggestion of the extent to which institutional factors and prevailing ideological views about Black women contribute to early motherhood and welfare dependency. Patricia Hill Collins suggests that Moynihan's theory uses Black women's performance as mothers to explain Black economic subordination.[6] As I see it, Moynihan's theory works in the reverse: Black economic subordination contributes significantly to Black mothers' performance.

With regard to Black teenage mothers, Moynihan's culture-of-poverty argument has effectively created racial divisions among teenagers by separating poor Black teenagers from middle-class White teenagers and so-called morally corrupt Black teenage mothers from all other adolescents. Equally important, the culture-of-poverty perspective reinforces gender inequality by focusing on the sexual life of teenage mothers, not on that of teenage fathers.

In a sense, the attempts of the culture-of-poverty theory to link teenage sexual behavior with Black cultural values puts a twist on social reproduction theory. In brief, this theory holds that societal institutions reproduce the social relationships and attitudes needed to sustain the existing relations of production in a capitalist society.[7] In the culture-of-poverty rendition, the institution of single-mother families reproduces attitudes, behaviors, and values permitting teenage sexual promiscuity and sustaining the nonrelationship with capitalism, that is, the reliance on welfare. Seen as a social deviant, the Black teenage girl reproduces more of her kind—a slap in the face of America's "family values." Ironically, the idea that these girls reproduce other "deviants" works to the advantage of a capitalist system, upholding the notion that society need not take any responsibility for those perceived to be unproductive and affirming that those who, for whatever reason, do not stand up for the status quo value system will find few seats reserved for them in the economic marketplace.

Moynihan's culture-of-poverty thesis, written more than thirty years ago, remains a powerful political theme today as politicians use the image of Black teenage mothers to provoke voters. In 1993 Governor Tommie Thompson of Wisconsin proposed a bill that would guarantee teenage welfare mothers eighty dollars a month in benefits if they married the fathers of their babies. After all, the proponents of the bill claimed, children of two-parent families do better than children of single-parent welfare families—"that's the American way." When that bill did not engender much support, Thompson urged voters in his state to vote against welfare supplements for unmarried teenage mothers. In 1996 a *New York Times* article focusing on the current economic trends reported that "teenage childbearing cost the taxpayer $8.9 billion a year." Douglas Besharov, a resident scholar at the politically conservative American Enterprise Institute, observed about the report, "A married teen-age mother is less likely to go on welfare." The culture-of-poverty thesis was also used by Tipton, Indiana, when the town's people discovered that "unwed teenagers accounted for 11.8 percent of births in Tipton county—a rate slightly higher than both Indiana's and the nation's." After much soul-searching, in a town where "football moms throw spaghetti dinners for the high school team," the mayor decided that the solution to teenage pregnancy was to challenge the values of these teenagers and to "bring back the stigma to teen sex and teen pregnancy," making the point that it is easy to inflame the minds of American voters with images of sexually free teenage girls copulating indiscriminately, dropping babies at every turn, and spending their days watching television, and thus destroying the texture of their community.[8]

The Economic Determinist Perspective

In recent years many theorists have moved away from the culture-of-poverty thesis to one that links the plight of Black teenage mothers to changes in America's economy during the 1970s and 1980s. They attempt to move from the culture-of-poverty focus on deviant Black families headed by women to families besieged by economic problems. Economic determinists take as their jumping-off point the structural requirements of the capitalist economic system and attempt to show that people reproduce their class situation. This thesis maintains that the economic changes brought about by the shift from an industrial to an information and service economy created enormous problems for Black families. William J. Wilson's groundbreaking study *The Truly Disadvantaged* shows that although economic advances during the 1960s enabled some Black families to leave the ghetto and its poverty as they became middle class, they left behind a community racked by poverty, unemployment, and poor Black families, mostly headed by women who were too impoverished to make it out of the ghetto. Many children in those poor families still see no way out of the despair that surround them. As economic determinists observe, people's sense of their lives is mitigated by their structural circumstances.[9]

In 1986 Leon Dash used the theme of limited options in his study of Black teenage mothers who lived in a poor section of Washington, D.C. The teenage mothers Dash studied knew about birth control and the consequences of sex without contraceptives but refused to use birth control. They wanted to become pregnant because they saw no future for themselves; they were neither scheming sexual monsters nor helpless leaves in a windstorm. Still, while Dash's study shows teenage mothers actively making decisions about their lives, it does not fully explain the experiences of Black teenage mothers.[10]

De Vonya Smalls's comments provided in the Introduction certainly support Dash's finding that teen mothers think motherhood gives meaning to the lives of girls who have few options. All the same, Dash's conclusions trouble me, with their underlying double standard, which holds girls, not boys, responsible for knowing about and using birth control while ignoring numerous studies that show most poor Black teenage girls do not receive sufficient sex education or birth control information.[11]

The Cultural Strategies Perspective

Carol Stack's ethnographic study *All Our Kin* has become a classic thesis about poor Black families. Stack's intention was to explore in depth the complex social world in which Black families survive. When Stack made her visits to the Black community in the 1970s, she saw Black families using an extensive network of kin and non-kin to help them through hard times. Her perspective is similar to Moynihan's in focusing on the cultural aspect of Black family life, but it differs by seeing these family networks as creative strategies for coping with oppressive economic conditions.[12]

Stack concludes her study with the observation that "the harsh economic conditions of poverty force people to return to proven strategies for survival." Much of what Stack saw in the 1970s had changed by the 1980s, when I heard these teen mothers talk about their lives. Stack asserts that the "child getting and child keeping" strategies she saw were all part of a unique Black culture.[13] I also saw "child getting and child keeping" as strategies, but they are not part of a cultural mandate; rather, they are an outcome of gender, racial, and economic inequalities.

Gender, Race, and Class Perspective

Why are so many Black girls barely past preadolescence having babies? This book intends to delve beneath the stereotypes of teenage motherhood and reveal the motivations, concerns, and strategies that make the lives of these young girls comprehensible. Let us take another look at two primary theories accounting for Black teenage pregnancies. Wilson's analysis of America's economic climate has made us understand the relationship between the collapse of the industrial economic structure and the plight of Black men and the Black community. To sociologists, Wilson's economic theory explains the conditions suffered by the Black community: they are the result of "the problem of male joblessness." Wilson argues that male joblessness is the single most important factor underlying the rise in unwed mothers among poor Black women.[14] However, because Wilson does not use a gender analysis, he takes into account neither women's employment problems nor how economic changes affect men's and women's relationships with each other.

Further, we must ask ourselves, How do children feel about their mothers and fathers if these adults are supposed to protect them from hunger and pain and fail to do so? How do women feel when they have to provide emotional support to their families but are so overworked that they cannot summon enough energy to do all they are supposed to do as mothers? How do teenage girls feel when their fathers leave them, for whatever reason, or when their mothers are overextended, or when teenage boys impregnate them and then abandon them? These questions are not considered in Wilson's analysis of Black lives.

Like Wilson's economic determinist theory, Stack's cultural strategies theory also looks at these problems of Black teenage mothers through a single lens. In acknowledging that the problems are basically economic, Stack is agreeing with Wilson, but she contends that Black families overcome these problems by using extensive family networks.

In addition to viewing the difficulties confronting the Black community only economically, Wilson and Stack assume that pregnant Black teenage girls have to contend only with being mothers. Black teenage mothers' experiences beg for a more complex analysis, one that encompasses the dimensions of gender, race, and class. For example, both Wilson's and Stack's theories ignore how Black teenage girls struggle with the adolescent process at the same time they are becoming mothers, and how these girls attempt to make sense of their lives on the basis of mostly erroneous information about themselves. Because they have faulty information, especially concerning sexual matters, and because they attempt to live according to family value models, these girls act on distorted views, creating even more difficulties for themselves, which they take into their adult lives.

In considering the causes of Black adolescent girls' problems, we cannot ignore the work of Carol Gilligan. As she describes in *Making Connections,* adolescence is a time of suppression as well as connection for girls. Girls of ages eleven and twelve can become unable to express themselves and can thus lose connection with others. During preadolescence girls exhibit self-confidence and assertiveness. Once they reach adolescence, their self-confidence diminishes. For example, they regularly preface their observations with the comment "I don't know," which Gilligan takes as a sign of repression. Other studies suggest that girls who lose their confidence also have lower test scores and school grades. These girls tend to focus on sexual relationships.[15]

During adolescence girls become concerned with reaching out to others and finding ways to develop trust in others. As Gilligan puts it, "The issue of holding together self and other—what has been called here the caring for the self as well as caring for others—may be a special issue of development during adolescence for some girls. The special vulnerability may be in finding a way of caring for the self while maintaining connections with others."[16] While Gilligan promotes the need to develop trust, she does not explain how race and economic factors influence girls' adolescent experiences. Therefore we do not learn how problems associated with race, such as living in a racially segregated community where many adolescents find being part of a gang the only satisfying activity they have at their age, can condition girls' adolescent experiences. Nor do we learn from Gilligan what it means for poor or working-class girls to lose their "voice."

Wilson's economic determinist theory, Stack's cultural strategies theory, and Gilligan's theory of girls' repressed adolescence contribute to our understanding of Black adolescent girls. However, such understanding is limited because each of these theories is from a single point of view. What is begging for our attention is the fact that adolescence is a time when Black girls, striving for maturity, lose the support of others in three significant ways. First, they are abandoned by the educational system; second, they become mere sexual accompanists for boys and men; third, these problems create a split between the girls and their families and significant others. What is needed to understand the losses, the stresses, and the large and small violences that render such teenage girls incapable of successfully completing their adolescent tasks is a gender, race, and class analysis, which is at the heart of this book. When early motherhood is added to these challenges, they become insurmountable. The adolescent mothers I saw were deprived of every resource needed for any human being to function well in our society: education, jobs, food, medical care, a secure place to live, love and respect, the ability to securely connect with others. In addition, these girls were silenced by the insidious and insistent stereotyping of them as promiscuous and aberrant teenage girls.

We must move away from these stereotypes and consider the ramifications of so much loss on the lives of Black adolescent girls. Patricia Hill Collins has called for an articulation of emerging "patterns of institutional oppression that differentially" affect Black women.[17] Following Collins's lead, I want to explore, further than Wilson and Stack have, those patterns of institutional oppression by asking some pivotal questions. What happens to interpersonal relationships when adolescent girls and their families have to deal with teenage pregnancy and motherhood? How do adolescent girls and their families feel about the indignity of having to call on others for the economic, emotional, and spiritual resources they require and having to look to the very people who will judge them stereotypically? What kinds of strategies do they develop to compensate for the loss of basic resources?

What I propose here is a theory of the poverty of relationships, a theory I have arrived at from a deepening knowledge of teenage mothers. Institutional oppressions do occur, and they are played out in a relational framework in which girls develop intentional strategies to form and sustain relationships with their significant others. These teenage mothers describe being disconnected from primary family relations, abandoned by their schools and by the men in their lives, and isolated from relations with other teenagers at the time of adolescence, when it is most important that they experience positive relationships. These teen mothers developed their strategies to make up for the poverty of their relationships.

The Destruction of Community Life

The lives of these Black teen girls are conditioned by the economic and relational changes that have occurred in the Black community in the last several decades. It is therefore necessary to highlight those changes so that we can truly understand their lives before and after they became teenage mothers.

During the 1950s and 1960s most Black families lived in fairly stable neighborhoods where families stayed for years. They lived ordinary lives, as ordinary as poor people's lives can be. Wilson describes these communities of the 1950s as places where Blacks did not hesitate to sleep in parks during the summer and Whites visited their taverns and nightclubs. There was a sense of strong family tradition in Black communities.[18]

In those days, fathers and mothers worked, loved, and had babies. Children played and slept in cold and cramped apartments. They played stoopball, double Dutch, red rover, ring-a-lievo, and hide-and-seek, singing in innocent voices, "One, two, button my shoe." Some kids were poorer than others, but they thought they were pretty much the same as the other kids on the block.

The streets of the Black community were very much like those of a small town. Everyone knew everyone else, or at least knew about them. This kind of knowledge was passed on by "old women" who spent much of their time gossiping about neighbors. Elijah Anderson

writes about "old women" like these. He calls them an "important
source of social control and organization for the community." These
women operated through bonds of kinship and friendship. They were
the ones others could "talk to" or "lean on," and they would dispense
advice, discipline, and corporal punishment, often filling an important fictive kinship role of extra parent or surrogate mother.[19]

These old women had an enormous influence on the community:
they were its conscience and its moral voice. Sitting on their front
steps, they would discuss the moral character of all the local
girls—who had it, and who did not. These old women knew all the
news: who was getting married, who was working or unemployed,
who was on welfare and why. If a teenage girl became pregnant, they
called her a whore, a girl who had loose morals, a daughter who had
had no proper upbringing. They would not hesitate to confront and
dress down girls who did not live up to their moral code: "What a
shame!" "A disgrace to the family!"

To the old women's way of thinking, girls were either good or bad.
If the girl did not steal, was not truant from school, and did not have a
baby before marriage, she was a good girl. Bad girls were deviants—people who, in the eyes of society, have "engaged in some
kind of collective denial of the social order," as Erving Goffman puts
it. Such people are viewed by society as failing to take advantage of
"available opportunities" and lacking respect for traditional values.[20]

I often think about those old women when people accuse the Black
community of condoning teenage pregnancy. It is just not true. Pregnant teenage girls were considered deviants in the past and are still
considered so today by many in the Black community.

Perhaps someone could have looked at the issue of Black teenage
pregnancies then to make predictions about the soaring birth rate
among Black teenage girls, which was two to three times higher than
that among White teenage girls during the 1960s, 1970s, and 1980s.
Back then, no one noticed the beginning of the trend.

Gangs, Drugs, and Family Disruption

During the 1960s the American economy underwent shifts that had a
drastic impact on poor Black ghettos. In most cities depression in

manufacturing sent people looking for work. These "old labor" industries, until then a mainstay for Black males (of whom over half were
blue-collar workers in the 1960s), were being replaced by industries
geared toward a service economy. Small businesses and plants that
formerly hired low-skilled or semiskilled Black workers went out of
business, left the cities to find cheap labor abroad, or hired White
women and recently arrived immigrants.[21]

By the mid 1970s the workforce changes had slammed Black neighborhoods hard. Men who did construction work were laid off. Mom-
and-pop stores, mostly owned by Italian or Jewish immigrant families, folded or moved away. These stores had employed many people
in the neighborhood and let families run up daily bills for essentials
like bread and milk, so their departure left a devastating void. Most
Blacks who remained in the community had no capital with which to
buy them.

During the 1960s and early 1970s apartment buildings were rapidly
being replaced by large, densely populated housing projects. The extreme crowding brought changes in space and material conditions—what Terry Williams and William Kornblum in *Growing Up
Poor* call our "community ecology." Williams and Kornblum make
clear the importance of community ecology on a person's life: "The
ecological features of the neighborhood establish the boundaries of
daily life. Jobs and small work assignments in the neighborhood may
offer young people their first earnings. The places to hang out, to com-
pete in athletics, to mark off as turf to be defended against outsiders—these are features of the local ecology that play a significant
role in the paths young people take to maturity."[22]

What is the community ecology of the poor inner city like? Richard
B. Freeman and Harry J. Holzer's analysis of data from the National
Bureau of Economic Research survey of Black youth ages sixteen to
twenty-four revealed that "Black youth living in the poorest areas of
inner cities were much more likely to be unemployed and less likely
to be employed than White youths or all black youths. . . . One-third
of them live in public housing; almost one-half of them have a family
member on welfare."[23] Only 28 percent of them have an adult man in
their household. The economic and social changes of the 1960s and
1970s brought havoc to the communities' ecology: gangs began to ap-

pear on the streets, bringing with them violence and drugs. Places to hang out, find jobs, or play safely slowly disappeared.

By the end of the 1970s, Black women and their families were also falling victim to these structural changes.[24] During the 1970s and 1980s the number of Black single-parent households steadily climbed upward from a low of 25 percent to reach 33 percent.[25] These single mothers were working at low-income domestic jobs, trying to support their families on five dollars an hour. By 1985 over half of all Black families were headed by women, mostly poor (the number of households headed by White women had climbed also, but not quite as quickly or as high: from 9 percent in the early 1970s to 18 percent by 1985). The majority of these Black women were forced to raise their children on poverty-level wages, earning little more than ten thousand dollars a year for a family of four.[26]

Two Communities: Oakland and Richmond

By 1986, the year I made my way into the heavily populated Black communities of East Oakland and Richmond, California, neighborhood life had nearly lost its vitality. These two communities had had a more promising beginning.[27] In 1860 thirty-one free Black adults and ten children arrived in the East Bay. They found work as laborers and farmhands in Oakland, the East Bay's first large frontier town. The new arrivals were allowed some freedom from the strict employment and housing segregation that Blacks generally experienced in more established cities in the United States, since Oaklanders were more concerned with developing the area than with applying racist policies. To avoid White-controlled institutions, Blacks established a private school for Black children and the first all-Black church in the United States, an African Methodist Episcopal mission. Several Blacks managed to buy choice real estate lots and prospered from their real estate holdings. By the end of the 1860s, Oakland had a stable community of fifty-five Black families, who were becoming increasingly prosperous.[28]

In 1869 the East Bay was transformed from a "chance stopping place" for Blacks seeking a better future into a compelling destination for migration when the Central Pacific (later Southern Pacific) Railroad chose Oakland as the western terminus of its transcontinental route. When the Pullman Company introduced sleeping cars for long-distance travel, it hired Black porters to provide personal services for passengers. By the end of the 1800s, Oakland and the smaller community of Richmond, the last stops on the railroad line, had become home base for the growing number of Pullman porters and their families. Later the railroad hired other Blacks to work as cooks, baggage handlers, waiters, and laborers in the passenger and freight depots. Eventually railroad workers required to live west of Adeline Street in order to be on call for unscheduled duty bought their own homes. In 1894 the first Black professional, a graduate of Howard University, arrived in the East Bay. He was soon followed by others who wanted the opportunity to work in an area that was quickly becoming an important Black community.

By the early 1900s Oakland and Richmond were vibrant Black middle-class communities of professionals and government workers. Black children from the Lake Merritt area of West Oakland attended private schools. Their parents bought property in new neighborhoods that stressed a "city beautiful" community and established a Black high society that attended formal balls and dinners and other elaborate social events. By the 1920s the success of these cities began to attract large numbers of southern Blacks, who came in search of jobs in construction and ship building. According to one resident, "Some didn't even have luggage; they could come with boxes, with three or four children with no place to stay." People who did not find housing crowded into any available space. Some old houses became occupied by as many as fifty people.[29]

The Great Depression brought Oakland's economic expansion to an end. Many in these two communities lost their jobs and were forced to seek public assistance for the first time, and at a rate four times that of Whites. Despite these economic hardships, Oakland's Black community tried to sustain a culture of art and music by launching art exhibits at the Oakland Art Gallery.[30] By the 1940s, when other Americans were pulling out of the depression, the percentage of unemployed Blacks in the Oakland community was six times their percentage of the population.

Between 1942 and 1945 war industries brought over fifty thousand Blacks to the East Bay. Most moved into Oakland to find jobs at

shipyards in Richmond. By 1949, overwhelmed by the large number
of Blacks seeking shelter, West Oakland had been declared a "blighted
area." Oakland's population grew from 8,462 in 1940 to 37,327 in 1945
and 47,563 in 1950. Richmond's grew from a mere 270 in 1940 to
14,000 in 1950. By the 1950s these communities had grown by ten
thousand people, causing one Oaklander to remark, "We'd go down
to Sixteenth Street station after school to watch people get off the
train and it was like a parade."[31] In 1954 the Oakland Citizens Committee for Urban Renewal endorsed the two-acre Acorn renewal project. In this effort to upgrade a district close to the downtown center
(convenient for shopping at large department stores), more than three
hundred buildings were demolished and nine thousand people were
forced to move. Because of housing discrimination, Blacks were not
free to move into the greater Oakland and Richmond communities;
instead, they had to move to newly available housing in East Oakland
and parts of Richmond. But in doing so they left behind churches,
political and entertainment clubs, and health care facilities, the very
community organizations that had given them support.

In Richmond, Black families living in small apartments or bunga-
lows tried to accommodate some of these displaced families by taking
them in as boarders. Families who did not receive such help had to
make do with trailers, shanties, and tents, seeming to fill every open
space. Despite these housing problems, Blacks were still moving into
these areas, hoping to take part in the employment opportunities offered by Ford Motor Company, the Mare Island naval base, the construction industry, and the significant Black culture. The Black population in Richmond, a smaller community, increased from 13,000 in
1950 to slightly more than 14,000 in 1960. The Black population in
Oakland, however, surged upward from 48,000 in 1950 to almost
84,000 in the 1960s. By the end of the 1960s, the tradition of Oakland's
and Richmond's middle-class gentility had all but disappeared.[32]

By the 1970s the Black communities of Oakland and Richmond
had experienced tremendous changes.[33] The destruction of the established Black community in West Oakland had forced Blacks to move
into East Oakland, where the structure of support and community organizations was lacking. These communities became plagued with a
number of problems: high unemployment, inadequate schools, crime-

and drug-related violence, and a growing number of teenage pregnancies. During the 1970s and 1980s, while Black families in Oakland
and Richmond were experiencing these tremendous problems and
the poverty of many Black families was becoming a focus of national
concern, the Reagan and Bush administrations cut government funding for housing, welfare, and educational programs. The government
funding cuts called for deep reductions in education, child nutrition,
housing assistance, and urban development grants.[34]

In 1986 I walked through East Oakland's and downtown Richmond's streets on my way to interview teenage mothers. It was hard
to believe these two communities were once thriving and middle-
class. Oakland and Richmond were a long way from the potential they
had held as a strong economic and social base for the Black settlers.
Now all I saw around me was the effects of poverty: deteriorating
housing, dilapidated public school buildings, and large numbers of
unemployed people. West Oakland now had more city housing projects (Acorn, Apollo, Morh) than any other neighborhood. In East
Oakland, Fourteenth Street and Fruitvale divided up flatland neighborhoods into small grids of single-family homes in various states of
disrepair and forbidding apartment complexes. These developments
included winding streets along their eastern edge and pockets of
greenery, but there was an unmistakable absence of community centers (except for churches) and stores and other local businesses offering job opportunities.[35]

The absence of jobs in Oakland and Richmond contributed to the
lowest median household income of any area, a little over ten thousand dollars in 1986.[36] The residents, many of them elderly, were
without cars. They had to walk across the freeway to services and
local government offices in the downtown area. Their situation was
in stark contrast to the prosperity once enjoyed when shipbuilding
jobs brought so many Blacks to Oakland from Texas and Louisiana.
Like that of many rust-belt cities of the Midwest and the East, Oakland's working population was left without local employment possibilities when manufacturing plants went out of business. Oakland's
high unemployment created a climate ripe for a host of criminal activities. As author Claude Brown put it when he revisited his old
neighborhood, "The streets had grown meaner," because of the

increased drug trafficking and violence.[37] Seldom did I see children playing on the streets with the air of abandon we had in New York two decades earlier. Instead, large groups of teenagers and older men lounged in front of the brick tower projects, some openly selling drugs.

Economic displacement and high numbers of single-parent households often appear together in the same community. So it was not surprising to find that in the same year I walked through those streets to interview the teen mothers, the city of Oakland reported that "close to 90 percent" of the families headed by women in Oakland were "living in poverty and receiving AFDC assistance."[38]

The living conditions of the teen mothers I interviewed support William J. Wilson's findings about socially isolated people in the Chicago city projects. Some teen mothers I saw were living in segregated communities of women-headed households. Oakland's city council acknowledged that 40 percent of these families were living in "neighborhoods where virtually all single mothers receive welfare aid."[39] The buildings, lacking care, had poorly lit hallways running maze-like around the apartment doors; graffiti proclaimed ownership of the walls; and weeds ran up the garden paths. Many of the teen mothers had poor educational skills and few prospects for stable employment. Others were educated and employed but still felt left out of the mainstream American community. This group of socially isolated families was growing fast.

In 1988, when the Crips and Bloods, two notorious gangs, were killing each other on Oakland streets, almost 73 percent of that city's Black teenage girls had babies, giving Oakland the dubious distinction of being ranked number 30 out of 108 large cities in the United States with a high percentage of births to women younger than twenty years old. The people of Richmond, a smaller community, could not make that claim, but they were watching the numbers with trepidation. Most of their teenage girls had never left their neighborhoods, attended a school dance, or gone unescorted to a movie.[40]

Few people, let alone old women, sat on the steps in front of their homes watching community life as they had done in my childhood. They were sitting indoors behind drawn window shades, deep frowns on their faces, lips pressed tightly together. They worried about drug dealers and crack-house landlords. When I talked about those earlier neighborhoods to seventy-year-old Annie Mae Jackson, she informed me that her community now was different: "Honey, now I gon' keep my butt inside." She was proud of being an active member of the Take Your Block Back from Drug Dealers Committee.

A few houses down the street, Carrie Evans, a stern-faced forty-year-old grandmother, addressed other concerns. She was in despair over raising the children of her teenage daughter, who had died from smoking crack cocaine: "I didn't think I would be doing this at this time of my life." Recently, a single mother had called me from New York City to tell me that her sixteen-year-old daughter was pregnant. A few months later a friend living in Oakland called to tell me that her fifteen-year-old daughter was pregnant. Another woman I knew told me that her seventeen-year-old daughter had died of a drug overdose. She had taken on the responsibility of raising her grand-child, something she was not prepared to do and deeply resented. These women were upset. How could their "little girls" do "such an awful thing?"

Others I talked to were equally perplexed about the number of Black teenage mothers who did "such an awful thing." Alma Sweets, a teacher in Oakland high schools for close to twenty years, ex-pressed her increasing frustration with the large number of teenage girls showing up in class pregnant: "How can you explain this? Surely, today's teenagers are more enlightened than twenty years ago. Don't they know more about sexuality issues and birth control today?"

All these social ills—unemployment, poor housing, gangs, drugs, disrupted families—contribute to the environmental conditions I saw when I visited the teen mothers. Driving down the street, I saw the signs of despair—the graffiti taking over every available space, the drug dealers moving in murky shadows toward their next cus-tomer—and as the teen mothers let me in their homes, I saw the same narrowing of choices, the threat of hopelessness. These communities, along with increasing numbers of Black people in Chicago, Detroit, Washington, D.C., and New York, present a picture of radical gender, class, and racial exclusion.

Talking to Teen Mothers

I began my search to understand the rise in Black motherhood by
interviewing two teen mothers referred to me by friends. They came
to my house early one Saturday morning and stayed for three hours.
Although I had prepared a series of general questions, the young
women had so much more to say that I was compelled to create a
more extensive set. Next, the director of a local family planning center let me attend a teen parent meeting, where I left a letter of introduction inviting those who were interested in my project to contact me. These teen mothers referred me to others. Eventually, I
created a list of fifteen teen mothers.

The director of the family planning center also introduced me to
Mary Higgins, the director of the Alternative Center in East Oakland.
The Center operated with a grant from a large charity organization
that allowed it to develop outreach programs geared to the needs of
the local teenage population. These programs included an alternative
school, day care, self-esteem development, parenting skills training,
and personal counseling. Mary in turn introduced me to Ann Getty, a
counselor at the center. Through Ann I met Claudia Wilson, a counselor for the Richmond Youth Counseling program. A short time after
that meeting, I began to work as a volunteer consultant for the Alternative Center and to attend meetings with counselors and others who
visited the center.

Through my contacts at the center, in the autumn of 1985 I met
De Vonya Smalls and twenty of the sample of thirty-two teen mothers
(see Table 1) who participated in this study. The rest of my sample
was drawn from other contacts I made in a network of community
workers at the Richmond Youth Service Agency and through my work
as a volunteer consultant there. The youth agency's counselors introduced me to teenage mothers who lived in the downtown Richmond
area. As a consultant, I was able to talk extensively with the adolescents who took part in teen mother programs.

After several months of making contacts, losing some, and making
new ones, I was able to pull together the sample of thirty-two teenage
mothers. Of this sample, I "hung out" with a core group of seven teen
mothers for a period of seven months, including sixteen-year-old

De Vonya Smalls. The other six teen mothers who participated were sixteen-year-old Susan Carter, a mother of a two-month-old baby, who was living with her mother and sister in East Oakland; seventeen-year-old Shana Leeds, a mother with a nine-month-old baby, who was living with a family friend in downtown Richmond; and eighteen-year-old Terry Parks, a mother of a two-year-old, who was sharing her East Oakland apartment with twenty-year-old Dana Little and her five-year-old son. The group also included twenty-year-old Diane Harris, who had become pregnant at seventeen and within months had exchanged a middle-class lifestyle for that of a welfare mother and was now living in a run-down apartment in East Oakland; Lois Patterson, a twenty-seven-year-old mother of two and long-term welfare recipient, who was living with her extended family in a small, crowded house in East Oakland; and Evie Jenkins, a forty-three-year-old mother of two, who was living on monthly disability insurance in a housing project near downtown Richmond. Like Diane Harris, Evie lost her middle-class status when she became a teenage welfare mother at age seventeen.

I accompanied these women to the Alternative Center, to the welfare office, and to visits with their mothers. Some of the teen mothers could not find private places to talk, so we talked in the back seat of my car, over lunch or dinner in coffee shops, in a shopping mall, at teenage program meetings, or while moving boxes to a new apartment—in other words, anywhere they would let me join them.

Interviewing the teen mothers on a regular basis was difficult: they frequently moved, appointments were missed, telephones were disconnected. One day I tried to call five mothers about planned participant observation sessions only to find all their telephones disconnected. A few mothers were willing to be interviewed because they thought they would benefit in some way. One mother let me interview her because she thought I had access to housing and could get her an apartment. Another thought I would be able to get her into a teen parent program. A few mothers did not bother returning my telephone calls once they discovered I could not pay them.

I did not pay the teen mothers or the others for taking part in these interviews. In exchange for their information, I told the teen mothers about my own family, gave out information about welfare assistance and teen parent programs, and drove them to various stores. I helped De Vonya Smalls move into her first apartment. I went out with the teen mothers to eat Chinese food, shared takeout dinners, and bought potato chips and sodas for, so it seemed, everyone's sisters, brothers, and cousins. I was in some homes so often that the families began to treat me like a friend.

I found myself caught up in the teen mothers' lives more than I had planned. I was able to capture changes in their lives. I watched a teen mother break up with her baby's father. I witnessed De Vonya Smalls and Shana Leeds move in and out of three different homes. I saw Shana Leeds go through the process of applying for AFDC. I sat through long afternoons with Diane Harris discussing her baby's "womanizing" father, only to attend their wedding a few months later.

I also talked to everyone else I could, including the teen mothers' mothers, Black and White teenage girls who were not mothers, teachers, counselors, directors of teen programs, social workers, and Planned Parenthood counselors. Many have definite views about teenage mothers, some representing a more conservative voice than we usually hear in the Black community.

Sadly, most of the teen mothers' fathers and their babies' fathers were not involved in their lives in any significant way. The teen mothers' lack of knowledge about the babies' fathers' whereabouts made it impossible for me to interview the men. The few men who were still involved with the teen mothers refused to be interviewed. The best I could do was to observe some of the dynamics between two teen fathers and mothers.[41]

Personal Histories

The teen mothers' ages ranged from fourteen to forty-three. Seventeen of them were currently teen mothers (aged fourteen to nineteen), and fifteen were older women who had previously been teen mothers (aged twenty to forty-three). The presence of the two age groups enabled me to appreciate the dynamic quality and long-term effects of teenage pregnancy on the mothers. The current teen mothers brought to the study a "here and now" aspect: I witnessed some of the family drama as it unfolded. The older women brought a sense of history and their reflective skills; the problems of being a teenage mother did not disappear when the teenage mothers became adults. The older women's stories served two goals for this book: to show that the black community has a history of not condoning teenage motherhood, and to locate emerging problems within the structural changes of our society that have affected everyone in recent years. The stories revealed in Chapters 2 and 3 show that these teen mothers' lives are more complex, and sadder, than we previously thought.

As a group, the teen mothers' personal histories reveal both common and not so common patterns among teenage mothers. The youngest teen mother was fourteen and the oldest was eighteen at the time of their first pregnancies. Seventeen teen mothers were currently receiving welfare aid. But contrary to the commonly held assumption that welfare mothers beget welfare mothers, only five teen mothers reported that their families had been on welfare for longer than five years. Twenty-four of the teen mothers had grown up in families headed by a single mother—a common pattern among teenage mothers. Thirteen reported that their mothers had been teenage mothers. Unlike other studies that focus on poor teenage mothers, this study also included five middle-class and three working-class teenage mothers whose parents were teachers, civil service managers, or nursing assistants. Nine of the teen mothers were attending high school (of whom six were attending alternative high school). Several had taken college courses, and two had managed to obtain a college degree.[42]

Along with capturing an ethnographic snapshot of the seven teen mothers, I conducted semistructured interviews in which I asked all the teen mothers specific questions about their experiences before, during, and after their pregnancies. I asked questions about various common perceptions: the idea of passive and promiscuous teenage girls, the role of men in their lives, the notion of strong cultural support for their pregnancies, the concept of extended family support networks, and the idea that teenage mothers have babies in order to receive welfare aid. Each teenage mother was interviewed for two to two and one-half hours. I audiotaped and transcribed all of the interviews.

I transcribed the material verbatim except for names and other identifying markers, which were changed during the transcription. I coded each teen mother on background variables and patterns. I read and reread my fieldnotes, supporting documents, and relevant literature. For this book I chose those quotations that would best represent typical responses, overall categories, and major themes. I used quotations from the core sample of seven as well as from the larger sample of thirty-two to include a wide range of responses.

Whenever possible I have tried to capture the teen mothers' emotional responses to the questions or issues. Often a teen mother would express through a sigh or a laugh feelings about some issue that contradicted her verbal response. For instance, when Terry Parks laughed as she described her feelings about being on welfare, I added a note about her laughter because it indicated to me that she was embarrassed about the subject. Without that notation, I would not have been able to communicate the emotional intensity with which she said the word "welfare" as she talked about her welfare experiences.

Through the Ethnographic Lens

I use an ethnographic approach to provide an intricate picture of how gender and poverty dictate the lives of these young teenage mothers and how societal gender, race, and class struggles are played out at the personal level. An ethnographic approach can bridge the gap between the sociological discussion of field research and the actual field experience. Studying these women through the lens of ethnography helped me move the teen mothers' personal stories to an objective level of analysis. The ethnographic method allowed the teen mothers to express to me personal information that was close to the heart. The method also allowed me to bring these Black teenage mothers into sociology's purview, to better understand them as persons, to make their voices heard, and to make their lives important to the larger society. The interviews and observations show that Black teenage girls' experiences are structural and troublesome. At all times I have attempted to make these teen mothers' stories real and visible by presenting the teen mothers' own words with as little editing as possible and by revealing their own insights into the interlocking structures of gender, race, and class.[43]

The Insider Interviewer

I could not walk easily into some teen mothers' lives. Being close to the people being interviewed made me both pleased and tense. Being an insider—someone sharing the culture, community, ethnicity, or gender background of the study participants—has its advantages and disadvantages. When the interviewer can identify with the class and ethnic background of the person being interviewed, there is a greater chance of establishing rapport. The person will express a greater range of attitudes and opinions, especially when the opinions to be expressed are somewhat opposed to general public opinion. The situation is more complex when interviewees are asked to reveal information that may serve the researcher's interest but not that of the group involved. "Don't wash dirty linen in public," they remind the researcher.[44]

The most difficult questions I faced, as do most insider interviewers, had to do with the politics of doing interviews in my own community. As an insider I had to decide whether making certain issues public would benefit the group at the same time that it served my research goals. I imagine that these interviews will raise questions. How will the White community perceive Black families if I discuss the conflicts between teen mothers and their mothers, or fathers who refuse to support their children, or the heavy negative sanctioning of these teen mothers by some in the Black community? My work would be taken out of context, several people warned me.

Every Black researcher who works on issues pertaining to her or his community grapples with these questions. We think about the possibility that our findings may contradict what the Black community wants outsiders to know. Some researchers select nonthreatening topics. Others romanticize Black life despite the evidence that life is hard for those on the bottom. And others simply adopt a code of silence, taking a position similar to that of the Black college teacher who in another context made the point to me, "I'm socialized to bear my pain in silence and not go blabbing about my problems to White folks, let alone strangers."[45]

Being an insider did not help me gain the confidence of the teen mothers and others immediately. Most were suspicious of researchers. I lost a chance to interview one group of teen mothers involved in a special school project because the counselors who worked with them did not like the way a White male researcher had treated the teen mothers previously. Indeed, these teen mothers had the right to be suspicious. What these girls and women say about their lives can be used against them by public policy makers, since the Black community is often blamed for its own social and economic situations.

But overall, being a Black woman was helpful, because eventually the teen mothers, realizing we had much in common, stopped being suspicious of me and began to talk candidly of their lives. Occasionally I could not find a babysitter and had to bring my little boy along. I found my son's presence helped reduce the aloofness of my role as researcher and the powerlessness of the teens' position as interview subjects. I was surprised at how helpful my son was in breaking through the first awkward moments. We made him the topic of discussion—mothers can always compare child-care problems. His presence also helped me counter some of the teenagers' tendencies to deny problems. When I talked to De Vonya Smalls about my son's effects on my own schedule, like having to get up at five in the morning instead of at seven, she relaxed and told me about her efforts to study for a test while her baby cried for attention. She also admitted to doing poorly in school.

I decided to study these teenage mothers because Black teenage mothers are not going away, no matter how much we ignore, romanticize, or remain silent about their lives. I strongly disagree with approaches that let the group's code of silence supersede the need to understand the problems and issues of Black teenage mothers. That kind of false ideology only perpetuates the myths about Black teenage motherhood and causes researchers to neglect larger sociological issues or fail to ask pertinent questions about the lives of these mothers. In the name of racial pride, then, we essentially overlook how the larger society shares a great deal of responsibility for these problems. The only way to reduce the number of teenage pregnancies or to improve the lives of teenage mothers is to understand the societal causes by examining the realities of these girls' lives. The time had arrived, as Nate Hare put it, for an end to the unrealistic view of Black lives.[46]

Chapter Two

Tough Times

Susan Carter

I didn't know nothin' about nothin'.
Sixteen-year-old Marnie Martin

In the East Oakland neighborhood where sixteen-year-old Susan Carter lived with her two-month-old baby, her mother, and two sisters, there were no parks. Nor were there many supermarkets or movie theaters. Susan hung out with her friends at the East Oakland mall, a run-down shopping center peppered with fast-food stores, small clothing boutiques filled with trendy but inexpensive clothes, a Payless shoe store, and a popular video game arcade. Susan's family shared a small, neatly furnished two-bedroom apartment across the street from the mall. After the baby was born, Susan applied for AFDC, but her application was turned down when the welfare worker informed her that her mother's $1,100 monthly salary as a nursing assistant exceeded the maximum allowed families of four.

Tall and pretty, with large, almond-shaped eyes that flashed when she smiled, Susan was a curious mix of adolescent and adult. Sometimes she appeared to be much older than her years, almost worldly. The next moment, she was cute and giggly, an adolescent dressed in typical teenage gear: T-shirt and jeans. Often we talked as Susan pushed curly-haired Jarmella in her stroller as we walked around the neighborhood of tiny box-shaped single-family homes interrupted occasionally by three-story apartment buildings like Susan's.

27

I did not have to walk far down Susan's street to realize that few middle-class Black families lived in her neighborhood. Most middle-class families had retreated from these bleak surroundings to the Oakland hills or to upscale Piedmont. Their move out of this neighborhood was not unusual. Most people who grow up in such inner-city surroundings want better schools, more space, a backyard, and less density. "If my son grows up to be a knuckle-head, it won't be because I didn't expose him to other possibilities," one writer observed after moving out of his inner-city neighborhood.[1]

The Black middle-class flight to suburbia left only three kinds of "success" stories to serve as role models for those like Susan who stayed behind: the flashy drug dealer, the sports figure, and the larger-than-life show business entertainer. Susan mostly saw the drug dealers cruising through the "hood" in BMWs with gold trim. Sports personalities, such as Michael Jordan and Larry Holmes, occasionally appeared at the Oakland Coliseum sports arena. After the events, and before they flew off to another city, dressed in beautiful and expensive jogging suits, they gave out autographs as part of promotional stunts.

Those people, being rich and famous, were special to Susan, and their lives did not register with her as the kind she could someday achieve. Susan's observations about her own life were textured by her mother's negative messages and her own observations of her friends' employment and unemployment potentials. Two close friends had recently applied for welfare. Almost all of Susan's school friends were in some kind of trouble; a few were selling drugs or were involved in gangs. She did not want to go that route, she insisted, but it was hard for this teenager to think of other paths to take when all she saw were three compelling, yet negative or unrealistic, models—the exaggerated success of drug dealers or sports or entertainment figures, compared with motherhood or work at McDonald's.

School Problems

Susan's story was hardly unique. Nor was the path that brought her to this place, the path she described as "coping with tough times." Susan told me about her school experiences one cool afternoon as we drove over to her high school, located in a predominantly Black school district noted for producing students with low test scores.[2] We parked in back of a square three-story brick building surrounded by a chain-link fence. On the other side of the fence, where a basketball lay between gum wrappers, dirty newspapers, and broken soda bottles, two boys were jumping up and down on a long wooden board.

Susan pointed to the darkened windows of her former classrooms: "I had English there, and Math in that one." School was "great" until the seventh grade, when Susan's classes became "boring and too easy," the teachers dull and uninspiring, and the work tedious. School was neither stimulating nor relevant. Most of the women she knew were working at low-level occupations or having children and, perhaps, getting married.

Susan did not get along with her teachers. Talking with her friends was easier than studying for classes. She began cutting classes to spend her days at the park with her friends talking about "this and that," and her school attendance "went downhill from there." "I wanted to go out with my friends," she told me. After a while most of her friends stopped coming to the park, but Susan stayed out of school anyway. Some days she fell asleep on the park bench. No matter how long and tedious the day was, she could not often bring herself to go back to school. By the end of the ninth grade, she was flunking most of her classes. "I didn't care." Her voice sounded convincing, but the "I don't care" attitude seemed like a front, hiding deep anxieties about herself and her ability to do well in school.[3]

Eventually Susan became passive and invisible when she was in the classroom. "I had to get out of school, just anything, to get out of school, something else besides school." She was bored. Susan did not consider transferring to another school. She began to believe she did not have the right attitude or motivation for school. Finally, two months after she learned she was pregnant, she dropped out of school—at the very age when school should have been a priority in her life.

Susan was similar to other Black Oakland students. According to an Oakland School District report, half of all Black students drop out of Oakland's schools. The dropout rates, always a problem, soared during the Reagan administration, when the school district suffered tremendous cutbacks. If children in Oakland's poor neighborhoods did manage to stay in school, one in five failed to complete basic courses in Math and English. Most of these children failed because their families did not have the economic and social resources to support adolescent children's academic performance.[4]

Bright, articulate, and yet bored, Susan did not blame the teachers or the school system. Why was school so difficult for her? Lacking her own explanation, she voiced the message of personal failure she had heard from those in authority. "It's all my fault." Everyone, including the school counselors, told her she was not working up to her potential. All she said in response was, "When I'm in class, it's like my mind stops working." She was convinced she should have worked harder. She brooded. "I must be lazy, because I'm not stupid. I can do the work."[5]

Several times Susan made the point that school was not for everyone. Anyway, she said a little defiantly, only a few of her classmates graduated from high school. To prove her point, she told me about seventeen-year-old Jean and sixteen-year-old Vicki, sisters who lived in an apartment upstairs. They had dropped out of school the previous year but seemed to be doing all right. Susan later admitted that Jean and Vicki were not finding work and were going to apply for welfare assistance. But Susan did not believe that a high school diploma was going to give her a better deal.[6]

Perhaps Susan and her teachers were right to blame Susan for a degree of her failure. But a number of studies show that teenage girls like Susan are taught to fail in school. In subtle and not so subtle ways, gender and race ideology operate in the class setting.

Michele Fine has explored the way gender ideology is reproduced in the high school experiences of 3,200 predominantly low-income Black students. The girls in her study tended to enroll in sex-typed vocational training courses, such as home economics, cosmetology, and secretarial programs, that teach skills for homemaking or jobs with low salaries and little life career advancement. Fine believes these girls accept this gender ideology because they do not have an alternative view of themselves.[7] They are often warned by their teachers, "You act like that, and you'll end up on welfare!" and encouraged to disparage the circumstances in which they live.

But Susan was missing out on more than just relevant school courses. In Susan's understanding of Jean's, Vicki's, or her own situation, it was not gender ideology that drove her out of school and made her seek refuge in the park or in intimate relationships. Susan lacked relationships with her teachers or other responsible adults in school, which would have enabled them and Susan to see beyond gender ideology and stereotypes about Black girls. Susan could not establish relationships with teachers and peers that would make school relevant. She only heard warnings from teachers that girls like her were prime candidates for poverty and welfare, so she could not see the importance of leaving the park bench.[8]

Susan spent most of her time avoiding school, partly because she was ignored, seemingly invisible in the classroom, and partly because the educational and cultural environment was so limited—there was no after-school program for Susan to attend since school funding was cut back. The cultural deprivation in Susan's school was appalling. What I saw at Susan's school confirmed Jonathan Kozol's insight that these schools are "extraordinarily unhappy places." Kozol, who has championed the rights of children for thirty years, writes, "[These schools] reminded me of 'garrisons' or 'outposts' in a foreign nation. The schools were marked frequently by signs that indicated DRUG-FREE ZONE. Their doors were guarded. Police sometimes patrolled the halls. The windows of the schools were often covered with steel grates." Kozol describes these Oakland schools as part of a "mainly nonwhite, poor and troubled system."[9]

These schools, plagued by violence, drugs, and gangs, reflect the drama in the world right outside the school door. "If you live to be thirty and not robbed, mugged, or drugged in this neighborhood, you're lucky," Susan grimly noted. Being surrounded by such an environment, school administrators focused on preserving law and order in their school yards, creating a prison atmosphere. Stern-faced school security guards stopped students to check their identification or room assignments.

School officials often blamed noisy and disruptive students for these school problems, but noise and chaos also seemed to be fostered by the teachers and administrators in the schools I observed. Authority figures barked orders over loudspeakers. At one school, where I had to sign in at the door after showing my identification to two burly guards, the principal and school staff interrupted class discussions, blasting their warnings over the loudspeaker: "If you are late, you must sign in at the first door; Mrs. Johnson's ten-thirty class will meet in room 234 for today only." At another school, a teenage mother informed me, a teacher kept a telephone on his desk, which rang frequently during the class hour.

The teachers and principal at one school I visited emphasized that students needed to learn "good" values. Some of the teachers interpreted those good values to mean gendered manners and attributes, which they passed off as graciousness and cleanliness. "Boys should remove their caps," a teacher informed me one day during my classroom visit, as she gave a teenager a demerit for wearing his cap in class. Another teacher told me she was impressed with the teen mothers, who "dress so neatly and brought their babies up so clean and neat." Yet a group of teen mothers bragged to me when I visited them at this same school that they received so little homework that they finished it during their forty-minute homeroom period.

The observation that the schools focus so much on teaching students "good" values and so little on teaching them how to put time and effort into their studies is striking not only because of the attitudes and values it discloses but also because it reveals the school environment in which Susan came to see only a few succeed. The path to success was too torturous for her to follow: "I couldn't read all that stuff in school, so I went to sleep." Her view was shared by other teen mothers. Education was not unimportant to these teen mothers. Most had been average to good students during their early school years. It was during adolescence that they began to drift away from school.[10] Although a few were still enthusiastic about education, most were like Susan, convinced by their own experiences and those of the people around them that education would not help them out of their situation. Susan's story, however, is much too complex to be explained by the lack of an adequate educational experience during adolescence or by the lack of opportunities. To understand why teenage Susan became a mother, we have to explore other factors as well.

Family Matters

When I asked Susan to talk about her personal life, she groaned. A sullen expression appeared on her moon-shaped face as she began to talk about her family. She was extremely angry at her mother. There had always been tension between them, and the hostility increased when Susan's mother realized she was expected to support her grandchild. Janet Carter, Susan's mother, had her own set of problems. Since he left, when Susan was young, Susan's father refused to pay child support and seldom visited the children. To make matters worse, Susan said, Janet Carter was experiencing problems at work. According to Susan, if her mother was not "bitchin'" about having to support her grandchild, she was grumbling "about her work and the long hours and the constant hassles with the patients and her supervisors."

Susan was sympathetic with her mother, who worked "like a dog," but she was also concerned because her mother's salary barely supported the family. Susan shook her head when I asked if her mother had other employment options. There was "nothing I can see"; most of the women she knew of her mother's age were on welfare, cleaned houses, or worked at McDonald's for $4.35 an hour. Susan's sympathy, however, only went so far. She believed her mother was not living up to her responsibility to love and support her daughter no matter what happened to her.

She blamed her mother for everything that had happened to her since her father had moved out. Until a few months before Susan became pregnant, her father occasionally visited the family or called his daughters to chat. Susan liked being with him. She recalled that when she stayed with him the summer she turned thirteen, he turned every occasion, like the nightly cookouts on the backyard grill, into a major event. That summer he found her a job typing letters and working on the computer at the local library. She was thrilled. On the next visit, everything changed:

We just didn't get along at all. I just was going out and getting drunk and I'd come home and I'd say everything to him. You know, all the things he did to my momma and all the things I hated him for when I was younger. 'Cause you know, he really hurt my momma a lot. I told him I hated him. I told him everything he deserved, and he didn't like me after that.

He did not like Susan's criticism one bit. He took her home and told her mother that he could not handle her. She could put Susan in a foster home for all he cared. She did not hear from him again until a year later, when she was eight months pregnant.

He called and, ah, I mean my aunt got a hold of him. And I told him I was pregnant. He was pretty shocked. And the only thing he said was, "Well, I guess I really need to talk to you." And he said he was thinking about coming down in two weeks, down to the Bay area. And, ah, he told me he'd call me back later on that night. And he, ah *(nervous voice),* never did. I never heard from him after that. I really don't know what he thinks about me because he never did say. He really *(low voice)* didn't say.

I think if my mother had stayed with my father and they would have talked to me and done a lot of things differently, I think I never would have gotten pregnant. I know I wouldn't have.

—Why not?

I know my father, he would never had let me. . . . I would have been too scared to try anything with guys, just too scared. 'Cause my mother, I knew anything I did, I could do anything I wanted. She wouldn't care. And if she would care, she couldn't help. See, that's another reason I got pregnant.

She felt her father's strong authority as head of the house would have been enough to save her from getting pregnant. Because her father was absent from her life, she had no one to hold responsible for the way it was turning out. "She didn't support me enough," Susan wanted me to know. The absent men were merely shadowy figures in the background of this teenage mother's life. Joney, the baby's father, was no help either, although he did promise Susan he would find a job and marry her as soon as he finished serving a two-year sentence for armed robbery.

Sexual Abuse: Uncle Freddy Dude

Susan was four years old when her uncle, who often baby-sat her, began sexually molesting her and his own three-year-old daughter. "He did it to me and my cousin Rachel." The molestation continued for four years:

And that's one thing I'll never understand my mom. She knew that he did that to me. My whole family knows, and he still lives with my grandmother, and he's still in the family. She doesn't pay attention. . . . In fact, she doesn't even like me any more, because . . . I don't know . . . I guess she thinks . . . I hate it. And my mom still lets him come over here just to fix the car. I tell her, "Mom, I don't want him over here." And she says, "Well, Susan, he's got to fix my car." You know, her car comes first.

—*Did she say anything to him?*

No, she never did. Never! And he came over here one time and we got into it. And he yelled at me. He can say anything he wants to me and she'll never stick up for me. Oh, that gets me so mad. I think, why would they do that? Why would they keep him in the family and stuff after what he did to me? If somebody did that to my daughter, I'd . . . I don't know what I'd do. I'd kill him.

—*Your daughter's here, and your uncle is still here. What are you going to do?*

I would never let him around her. I don't even want him around me. . . . I'll take her away. I'll just leave.

—*Do you think that there may be a connection between the molestation by your uncle and your early pregnancy?*

I don't know if that had anything to do with it. I know that after that I blocked it out. I know he was wrong. It just made me mad and I blocked it away. I just never wanted to think about it anymore. It didn't bother me after a while.

That is, she was not bothered until she began to have recurring dreams that stirred up her memories of the sexual abuse:

You know the Freddy dude from the movie *Nightmare on Elm Street?* I had a bad nightmare about him. There was this same house that my uncle molested us in. And Freddy had us locked up there. When I woke up, I was crying. I was shaking. And I jumped in bed with my sister. This was not long ago. Before I got pregnant, I guess. I was suppose to see a psychologist. It was all blocked up and it had to come out sometime. Those feelings are still there.

Susan's story of early childhood sexual abuse reveals a complex issue that does not lend itself to simple explanations. Some evidence suggests a connection between premature and harmful sexual experiences and teenage pregnancy. A study of 445 Black teenage mothers reports that more than 60 percent of them were forced to have an unwanted sexual experience at some time in their lives; one-third were younger than twelve at the time of the first forced experience. More than one-quarter reported that they were harassed by family members.[11]

Although the study does not directly link sexual abuse and teenage pregnancy, it does suggest that sexual abuse may make young girls feel tremendously vulnerable and dependent. When girls like Susan Carter are sexually abused at an early age, they may learn to define themselves and others primarily in sexual terms. The teen mothers I talked with reported having ongoing nightmares, problems in school, and problems with intercourse, which are symptoms displayed by sexually abused victims.[12]

For a number of reasons, sexual abuse may be the most critical event in a girl's young life. As they move toward independence, adolescent girls seek security in some kind of attachment to others. They are handling crucial developmental issues, such as adult connections, physical maturation, and where to place their trust. Sexually abused teenage girls, who have found their love and trust betrayed, may have little emotional energy left to invest in other areas of their lives, such as doing well in school, and so may lose interest in them, especially if they can expect little extrinsic or intrinsic reward.

Is Susan's experience an exception in this study? I asked other teen mothers questions about sexual abuse. Some said, "Absolutely not!" A few were vague: something may have happened, but they could not remember the details. Only twenty-six-year-old Tonya Banks, a stout and intense older teen mother, recalled being sexually abused by her uncle when she was eight years old.[13]

Many teen parent counselors at the Alternative Center, where I worked as a consultant, admitted hearing "a million stories" about sexual abuse. Some counselors believed these "stories" to be true; others were leery. Several believed that teen mothers had ulterior motives for their accusations: some may have been responding to the media's focus on sexual abuse, others looking for sympathetic attention.[14]

Jean Carroll, a teen parent program coordinator for the Oakland school district, raised her eyebrows when I asked whether she had data on sexual abuse. "Well, no. We don't really keep those kinds of reports." She did not know of any agencies with such records. She admitted, "We don't know how many cases, since the teen mothers may not tell us." According to this program coordinator, the staff of the parent programs could not keep records of these reports because it was committed to keeping the students' records confidential. It is ironic that this protective strategy allows a serious issue like sexual abuse to go unreported.[15]

Learning about Sexuality

Often during my visits with Susan, we would walk over to McDonald's to buy French fries, Susan's favorite food.[16] Several times a group of neighborhood teenage boys, lounging in front of the restaurant jostling with each other and slapping high fives, yelled, "I'm gonna git me some of that," when we walked past them. Susan would stare at the ground. One day a group of boys began jokingly to describe various sexual acts they wanted to perform on Susan. We made a hasty retreat. Susan was unnerved by the sexual harassment.

Michele Wallace describes the way men notice the physical development of a young girl such as Susan: "Some of the nice little old men who used to pat her on the head when she was a child begin to want to pat her on the ass when she is thirteen. The neighborhood pimps and hustlers begin to proposition her." Wallace contends that young girls (like Susan) are extremely vulnerable and are unprepared for the way men respond to their maturing bodies.[17]

Susan was typical of the other teenagers in this study in that she developed physical maturity early. The Black teenage participants of one study developed early signs of pubertal changes by age nine, with menarche coming at 12.5 years of age on the average. By the time they reached the age of thirteen or fourteen, these girls found themselves confronting teenage boys' sexual advances earlier than White girls.[18]

While Black teenagers may physically mature earlier than other teenagers, all teenagers are maturing faster than the women of their mothers' generation. For instance, two generations ago teenage girls did not have to decide whether to have sex, take drugs, or drink until they were older. Today they make these choices in junior high school. A generation ago teenagers pursued hobbies and same-sex relationships. Now boys and girls often interact in peer groups. Girls today reach menarche, the time when they become capable of conception and sexual activity, as early as ten years old. The majority of the young women in my sample began menstruation between the ages of eleven and thirteen. During their mothers' generation the average girl started her menstrual cycle at age thirteen.[19]

Missing from Susan's talk about sexuality was a well-defined attitude about her sexuality or about abortion: "We just didn't worry about that stuff. We never thought about it—getting pregnant, really getting pregnant." The myth that they could not get pregnant during their first sexual intercourse was very popular among the teen mothers.

The idea that teenagers do not understand their reproductive abilities may surprise some, but it is that very lack of knowledge—part of a general belief system holding that young girls do not need to know about their bodies—that rendered Susan and the other teen mothers largely ignorant about their sexuality: "I didn't really know nothin' about douching or about birth control."

Susan did not remember who told her about sex and sexuality, but she was sure it was not her mother: "My mother didn't tell me about menstruation until I had my period, and I almost died. Never! She didn't even wanna talk about it. My mother, she wouldn't talk to me to really let me know what this was." Most of the teenage mothers did not fully understand the menstrual cycle. Most did not acknowledge their first menstruation, although it signaled a major change in their lives. They did not make the connection between the start of menstruation and their ability to become pregnant.[20]

Nor did they discuss sexuality with their parents. Girls who did talk with their parents discussed dating and boyfriends but not sexual intercourse, morality, or birth control. Mostly, as Greer Litton Fox and others observe, teenage girls ask their mothers how to handle boyfriends on a date (prior to and not including sexual intercourse).[21] Despite the lack of communication about sexuality issues, the mothers of the teens kept close supervision of their daughters' menstruation cycles. Susan and many of the other teen mothers said their mothers questioned them consistently, recording their menstrual cycles on calendars every month. (Since these were self-reports, the teen mothers were able to keep the news of their missing monthly periods to themselves.)

Some of the teen mothers admitted they were curious about sex. Several tried to talk to their parents. Sixteen-year-old Marnie Martin recalled being a little frightened by her feelings and wanting to talk to her parents, but, "That was the problem! My parents didn't really talk to me about sex. They used to say that 'you couldn't really have sex.'" Marnie did find the courage to talk to her mother:

I think I was thirteen when I first started having sex. My best friend thought I was crazy, 'cause I went to my mother and said, "Well mom, I like this boy and I might be doing something with him and would you take me to get birth control?" And she said, "No, because once you start taking those pills you'll become sterile." See, I want kids. I love them and I want them. So it scared me. At the time the only thing I knew was condoms. I said no, I'm not going to mess with that. It wasn't as if she wasn't warned, because I came to her and asked. And my girlfriend said, "No, Marnie, that's a lie. I don't know why your mother said that."

Four teen mothers told me that their mothers fell back on what they had learned incorrectly from their own mothers. Tracy Alexander laughingly mimicked her mother's high-pitched voice: "You can get pregnant by kissing a boy." In a study on Black teenage mothers, Joyce Ladner has found that mothers pass on to their daughters the misinformation about sex and biological changes that their mothers had passed on to them. As Ellen Kisker notes, by using folk techniques and religious sanctions to limit information about sexuality, mothers not only misinform their daughters about sexuality but also impart their values. Marnie's mother did not approve of her daughter's desire to engage in sexual activity. But misinforming and scaring Marnie did not prevent her from becoming sexually active. Marnie's mother did not comprehend the importance of sexuality for her daughter.[22]

The parents of many of these teen mothers believed that telling their daughters about birth control could be interpreted as permitting them to have sex. Several of the teen mothers' mothers admitted that they did not know what to say to their daughters or how to be open and frank about sexuality. When Marlee Conners, a shy woman in her late thirties, said she had told her seventeen-year-old daughter Jasmine about birth control, Jasmine claimed, "This is all in her mind. She don't tell me a thing." De Lesha Simons, a seventeen-year-old mother, recalled a similar story: "My mother said, 'I told you that.' I said, 'Ma, what you told me wasn't enough to fill a shoe.' I guess she thought she had told me." Susan's mother, Janet, did tell her, when

Susan questioned her about sex, that she would learn more about it when she married.

Love at Fourteen

Susan met Joney Glover, a "cute" seventeen-year-old unemployed high school dropout, at a friend's party. He paid Susan a great deal of attention at the party, which she found very flattering. After that, they went everywhere together. Most of the teen mothers had similar stories—meeting the babies' fathers at parties or at school, where boys hung around the school yard. When an attractive girl crossed a boy's path, he gravitated to her very quickly, arranged for a meeting, and encouraged a friendship that became sexual in a short time. The "sexual hits"—the young mens' pickup strategies—pervaded these teenage mothers' stories. When the girls reached the ages of twelve and thirteen, they found the boys at school talking to them, walking them home, and telling them how cute they looked in whatever they wore.

Elizah Anderson argues that unprotected teenagers such as Susan from mother-only households, or those who do not have a strong male presence in the household, may be attracted to young men eagerly selling themselves as ready for commitment. When I raised this point with Susan, she quickly assured me that Joney had not pressured her into sexual involvement. Joney was, after all, an ordinary boy in Susan's eyes. But according to Anderson ordinary boys may be acting within a social context that allows them to develop the kind of sexual harassment that writer Michele Wallace recalls. The social context within which Black boys' sexual skills are developed consists of poverty, poor educational facilities, high unemployment, fatalistic attitudes, and the need to "prove" oneself through early sexual experimentation. The boys' attitude toward these girls is also consistent with the patriarchal view of women as sexual objects.[23]

Susan did not know how racism and sexism might affect Black men like Joney. All she knew was that when she turned thirteen her mother allowed her to stay out later than before. Her friends pressured her to drink, smoke pot, and have sex. "Everyone is doing it," they informed her. "So I had to go with the crowd, that's what it was." Joney began to pay attention to her: "He was coming to school all the time to meet me." She was "scared." She did not have the time to think through her feelings about sexuality, dating, or birth control: "When he asked me, I didn't know what to do. But I did it finally."[24]

Susan "did it," but sex did not have the erotic meaning usually associated with it: "It was disappointing. I regretted it afterward. I thought, God, is that all it is?" She laughed at the thought. I joined in the laughter because the other teen mothers had expressed similar feelings. Susan's question, "Is that all it is?" contradicted the common view that Black teenage girls have hot and shameless sex lives.

We adults often perceive the world of adolescents through our own steamy glasses. Sometimes, as Lillian Rubin so astutely notes, rather than wanting to have sexual relations, teenage girls may simply want to be kissed and caressed. According to Robert Cole and Geoffrey Stokes, teenagers differ from adults in their reasons for engaging in sexual activity: for teenagers like Susan (and perhaps Joney), sex may be a reprieve from "a life that can be, often enough, boring or demanding or puzzling."[25]

Cole and Stokes's observations made sense to me as I listened to Susan. In Susan's story I heard no words of hot desire or unbridled lust. Sex was a mechanical act, a way to release pent-up anxieties and tensions, as Cole and Stokes suggest, and perhaps an escape from her personal problems. This is not the view most have of teenage mothers' experiences. It would be easier to blame Susan, as so many others do, for letting this situation happen to her in the first place, but we must not overlook the environment in which Susan lives.

Elizah Anderson would not be surprised that Susan fell in love and became sexually involved with Joney. As Anderson notes, young Black women who face a bleak future, having only a limited education and few employment skills, may easily be captured by young men's whispered promises of "love forever."[26]

To add more complexity to Anderson's analysis, we have to understand that Susan did not think it was morally wrong to engage in sexual intercourse. Like many teenagers, Susan valued the spontaneity and romance of her relationship with Joney, which would have been compromised by planning for sex. Several teen mothers thought that having sex before marriage was a "sin" but admitted overcoming that belief when they fell in love, echoing Susan's comment: "For the first time, I was really in love. So we had sex."

Birth Control Knowledge

"Why didn't you use birth control?" I asked Susan. Despite Leon Dash's observation that the teenage mothers in his study were knowledgeable about contraception, Susan did not learn about birth control from her mother or anyone else. Several teen mothers I spoke with made the same claim as those in Dash's study, but in fact few knew about birth control or other issues regarding their sexuality. For example, none of the teen mothers could adequately discuss the man's role in reproduction. Only two were well informed about contraceptives.[27]

The use of contraceptives presents a dilemma to teenage girls. According to Kristen Luker, for the teenager to use contraceptives is an admission she is sexually active. If the teenage girl uses contraceptives, she loses all claim to spontaneity. If she buys contraceptives in the drugstore, she acknowledges in a fairly public place that she intends to have sex. Another part of the problem for teenagers is their ambivalence about norms governing their sexual behavior. Whose norms to follow—their peer group's or their parents'? How can they understand these norms, given that parents refuse to discuss them, other than to say, "You can't"?[28]

"Why didn't you take sex education classes in school?" I asked Susan. She wanted to take a course on sex education, she told me, but the school did not offer one. A few teen mothers said their schools did offer these classes, but they were not very helpful. Two teen mothers who attended their schools' sex education programs found them to be too clinical, the language too technical, the teacher too aloof, and the material too removed from their real experiences. In most cases these classes were held only one day during the semester. Marnie Martin was absent from school the day her class decided to discuss sex education material. By the time the next semester rolled around, she was pregnant and on welfare.

Why do so many teen mothers learn so little in sex education courses? The teen mothers were caught in the middle of the debate over what should be taught and whether the family or the school is responsible for teaching sex education to children. On one side of this debate are fundamentalists and many others who argue that young girls do not need to know about their sexuality and that such education in fact promotes promiscuity. This view has been contradicted by several studies conducted by the Alan Guttmacker Institute finding that education programs increase knowledge but do not lead to promiscuous behavior.[29]

The media also bear responsibility for poor sex education. According to Millicent Philliber, whose study criticizes the media's portrayal of sex and sexual attractiveness, the media often depict adults being carried away by sexual passion, but they do not show that passion leads to coitus, or that coitus leads to pregnancy.[30]

Sex education courses may prevent some, but not many, teenage pregnancies. But it is imperative that teenagers like Susan Carter receive accurate information about their sexuality through such courses for another reason as well. As Susan's comments show, and as other teen mothers' descriptions of their early years will demonstrate throughout this book, these adolescent girls learned at an early age that they were sexual, but they did not learn about sexuality in a way that would give them a positive sense of being women. Mainly, they experienced the mainstream gender ideology operating through the men they met in the school yard and through the school that refused to give them adequate information about themselves as women. According to this ideology, for example, a girl's successful transition into adulthood depends in large part on her ability to attract boys: therefore sexual naïveté is advantageous since a knowledgeable girl may be labeled as being "too smart for her own good," and only "bad" girls develop strategies about sexual activity (or about any other area in their lives except for being married and having babies).

Dumbing Down Sex Education

Susan told me about an egg experiment conducted in a former class in lieu of a formal sex education course. As a lesson to deter teen pregnancies, each student was given an egg to care for. They had to give the eggs names and think of them as their newborn babies. The teachers believed that the students would learn about the difficulties of raising children if they had to carry the eggs everywhere and not break them. At the end of the week, the students were to write reports on the responsibility of caring for their "babies." Before the week was over, however, some of the braver students grew tired of the experiment and decided to end it. They took turns rolling their eggs down the corridor yelling, "Crack, baby, crack." The school abandoned the egg experiment after the cracked eggs left a yellow mess on the hallway floor.

Neither the sex education courses nor the egg experiment taught Susan or the other teen girls how to handle the daily sexual advances of the adolescent boys and young men. Access to important information about their sexuality was denied them. Whatever information they could glean was restricted to vague abstractions; the time allocated to its teaching was minimal. Such sex education was ineffective in preventing Susan's pregnancy, let alone addressing the severe social problems that underlie the phenomenon of teenage pregnancy.

Baby's Love

It was late in the evening. Susan and I were comfortable with each other, sitting on the small sofa in the living room, our feet curled up under us. This would be my last visit to Susan's home, and I wanted to ask a few remaining questions.

—*Why do you think you got pregnant?*

Well, it wasn't planned.

—*Did he want you to have a baby before you got pregnant?*

It was unexpected.

—*Did you want to have your baby?*

Yeah.

I usually asked the teen mothers these questions several times, in different ways, throughout the course of our interviews. Often, I realized, they had not decided what they really thought about getting pregnant so young. It was usually during our final discussions that the teen mothers came to grips with their feelings about their pregnancies and about being teenage mothers. When I asked Susan again, she briefly paused before responding: "So . . . um, because it's . . . for a lot of reasons. I didn't want an abortion. I wanted my baby. I just thought . . . I guess I don't really know why *(high-pitched voice)* in some ways." This was the first time she admitted any feelings of confusion.

Susan and I continued our conversation:

—*Perhaps you want something from the baby that you didn't get growing up?*

Susan answered quickly:

Oh, love. She makes me happy. It's fun watching her grow.

—*Did you miss out on something when you were growing up?*

Oh yeah. My mother was too busy working and spending her time elsewhere to care very much about raising me.

Susan's comments tell us that she became pregnant in response to her feeling of alienation from her mother. The only way to handle that feeling was to give birth to a baby, thereby guaranteeing that she receive the love and security she needed. Those comments do not tell the whole story. She did not mention her own uncle's or father's role in this family drama. Nor did she mention how she felt taking classes she did not master. These important details were missing from her final comments, although they helped fill in the story of why fifteen-year-old Susan defied everyone's wish that she have an abortion and sought love and security in motherhood. She did talk about being proud of her relationship with Joney, the baby's father.

For the Love of Joney

Susan talked about Joney in glowing terms, calling him the "most supportive person in my life. He always gave me a lot of support." She informed me that Joney had "class": "He's not a lowlife. It's just that sometimes, his friends, they shoot up and they do crazy stuff." Joney had a history of doing "crazy stuff." She said in a low voice, "I kept telling him, you can't live like that 'cause it's going to catch up to you." It did catch up with him, and he was then serving time in a youth camp. But Susan was sure he would change. She felt confident that when he served his time, he would become the kind of man she wanted him to be. She expected he would find a job as a laborer on his release from the youth camp, because, as Susan put it, "He wants to make it so bad now, and settle down and marry me."

"Did he want the baby?" I wanted to know. Susan responded: "He came to me and said, 'Susan, don't carry my baby if you don't want to. 'Cause if you don't wanna keep it, just give it up for adoption. Whatever you do, that's okay.' He says a lot of things like that. He's so supportive." Susan and I read Joney's comments quite differently. Perhaps because he expressed his views in such negative terms, it struck me that in deciding to have this baby, Susan had taken on all the responsibility for the baby. I wondered what would happen to Susan and Jarmella if her relationship to Joney cooled. Would he hold her solely responsible for the baby's upbringing?

Susan settled back on the sofa. She began to talk quietly about Joney's other child: "He has a four-year-old son he doesn't know. He didn't care for the girl at all. Her mom called him up and said, 'My daughter's in the hospital having your baby.' And she expected him to do everything for her after that, but he couldn't. He never got over that. He never paid any attention to her. He still doesn't. The kid looks just like him. But he still wonders if the baby's really his. The girl, she's a tramp." Susan believed Joney was right to ignore the girl and the baby. After all, she reasoned, "He doesn't know if the baby is his," although the baby looks just like Joney. Susan insisted with an air of smugness that because the girl was a tramp, she deserved the kind of treatment Joney gave her. She was also sure that Joney would not treat her the same way; she reminded me of how "supportive" he had always been to her.

In some ways Susan's story was about the normal transitional process girls go through during adolescence, when they are learning to handle a changing physiology and the beginning of sexuality identity. In other ways it was about societal pressures, the inadequacy of the sex education being taught to Susan at home and at school, and the freer expression of sexuality she saw in the media and from the boys who were beginning to relate to her in a sexual way. She had no strategies to handle these developmental and social issues.

Having been taught almost nothing about relationships with young men, Susan had no decision-making skill that might help her discern Joney's poor judgments about his other baby and his lifestyle. At this stage of Susan's life, she was doing what adolescents do: she was basing an attachment on what she saw as Joney's trust and sensitivity. She did not find love and security in her family. Susan's reliance on Joney's support became crucial after her family failed to comprehend the nature of her alienation from school. She began to look for support elsewhere after she was sexually abused for four years by her uncle, after her family failed to take her charges against her uncle seriously, and after she began to have disturbing dreams about that experience.

It was also hard for Susan to navigate the world outside her door. She had no strategy to handle the complexities of growing up in an urban environment ruined by drugs, delinquency, and unemployment.

It is in Susan's description of developmental issues and school and family problems that I have gained a deeper insight into the poverty of these teen mothers' relationships.

Chapter Three

Her Baby Days Are Over

De Vonya Smalls

I'm just a regular old lady.

Fifteen-year-old Junie Grant

De Vonya was neatly stacking moving boxes at the front door of her friend's apartment when I drove up to the old frame house in East Oakland. She had moved out of her mother's house several weeks before because the tension between her and her mother had escalated since De Vonya's pregnancy and the birth of her baby. Since her friend needed the space for her own five children, she had to move again—her third move in three months. De Vonya did not have any transportation, so I offered my car. We loaded up the car and drove off to her new apartment in the Acorn housing complex.

De Vonya was in the eleventh grade, with plans to graduate at the end of the following school year. In contrast to Susan's pessimistic view of her education, De Vonya boasted of earning As and Bs in school, thinking they would lead her to the "good life." "I had some good classes. I had all college prep classes. You see, I was going the whole day." But De Vonya's plan was almost thwarted by a school counselor who informed her that it was in her interest to transfer to another school where she could take alternative classes geared to the needs of teenage mothers like her. "I ain't no fool," she told me. "Those are pregnancy schools where all they teach is courses on parenting. They just go half days. That's a lot of hours you be missin' learnin'."[1]

De Vonya laughed as she described what happened to her when the administrators at her current school learned about her pregnancy:

Yeah, they tried to kick me out. They told me I had to go to another school. I told them, "I ain't goin'." The vice principal sent me a letter. I tore that letter up and went to school the nine months. And every time I'd see the nurse, I'd just hide from her.

We both laughed.

—Why did the school officials want you to go to another school?

'Cause they feel that if you get hurt on the school's premises you can sue 'cause they don't allow pregnant girls. I think [you've] gotta leave [at] five months.

De Vonya had some support in her efforts to stay in school. Several of her teachers defied the school officials by letting her take classes. Her friends also helped her. If a school staff member happened to pass by while she was standing in a hallway, "[My friends] would tell me and I'd hide behind them or I would go out another door. Sometimes I'd hide in an empty classroom if none of my friends were around." She vowed to stay in "normal school." (The teen mothers often used such language, with its psychological meaning, to distinguish between the situation of a teen mother and that of other teenagers.) She had plans to "[go to] computer school or get into the police department."

De Vonya told no one, not even her mother, that the baby's father also attended her school. In fact, she did not talk about him at all: "He refused to claim the baby. . . . I just decided to leave him alone. So nobody'll know." She did not want to talk about Matthew with me. A few minutes later she relented. She met Matthew, a "cool, quiet" boy of her age, in a class. They were immediately attracted to each other and became sexually involved after a few movie dates. When he refused to speak to her after she became pregnant, she said, "I was mad at him." She was also confused by the way he treated her. She later described her relationship with Matthew in more detail. Nine months after their first sexual encounter, she missed her period. "It couldn't mean anything, I thought." Her mother thought otherwise.

[My mother] kinda figured, 'cause I was sleeping a lot. And then she said, "Well, I'm taking you to the doctor for a checkup." We went. My mother was in the other room with my sister when the doctor told me to come in the room. And I went into the room and he said, "You're pregnant. What are you going to do?" Tears were coming down out of my eyes. And the doctor said, "Do you want me to tell your mother while you're in here?"

I said, "No, let me leave and you tell her." I walked out the room and he told her and I hear her cry like, "No!" I said, "Oh, my God." And she had her belt. You know those big belts the girls be wearing? She had it in her hand and she had punched the doctor. I guess she was so angry. I didn't really talk to nobody. I was nervous. We had to walk home from the doctor, and she was mad. I could tell she was mad. I was walking real slow, my knees were shaking and my hands were sweatin'.

Later on she tried to convince me to have an abortion. I said no. And she called my father and was crying on the phone. And she called my aunt in Phoenix, and she was crying on the phone.

Several teen mothers had similar stories—their mothers found out about their pregnancies at the same time they did. But many of the teen mothers said they knew they were pregnant months before they told their mothers. They dreaded telling their mothers, because, as Carita Hughes put it, "I was scared. I didn't know what she would do." They all said they were so concerned about their mothers' reactions that they tried to hide their pregnancies as long as possible. Junie Grant, a fifteen-year-old teen mother, exemplifies this pattern: "I didn't show until I was six months, actually showing, sticking out. I kept it in. I got sick, so my mother took me to the hospital and they told her." Junie hid her bulging stomach from her mother for several months by wearing bulky sweaters. La Shana Lewis, another young mother-to-be, used the same ruse: "I wore real big clothes and lots of layers. And things in my pockets in the front. And that was a real turmoil for me because, just hiding it and not being able to breathe because something was so tight, you almost passed out."

The delay seemed to the girls to have the desired effect, for they controlled information about themselves by denying that they were pregnant. But the teen mothers paid a tremendous price for the postponements. They waited so long before telling their mothers that it was impossible for any of them to have an abortion. Only two of them received any kind of prenatal care. The Alternative Center, where I volunteered, was alarmed at the number of teen mothers who delayed reporting their pregnancies, and the Center attributed the high Black infant mortality rate to the teen mothers' refusal to admit that they were pregnant.[2] One of the Center's pamphlets warned the teen mothers: "Don't Bury Your Head in the Sand [by saying,] 'My period is late because I've been upset . . . I've been upset because my period is late,' or 'Maybe I'll get my period next week.'"

Daughters and Mothers

During the drive to her new apartment, De Vonya and I had the chance to talk about her relationship with her mother. Since twenty-four of the teen mothers were from single-mother households and their primary relationships were with their mothers, I wanted to know what impact, if any, the teenagers' pregnancies had on these relationships. What happened in De Vonya's family when she became pregnant and had to rely on her mother as her only available support? What kind of support did she receive from her mother before, during, and after her pregnancy? De Vonya fed her baby, gave her a bottle of water, and nestled her snugly in her arms as we sped along bustling East Oakland streets. When I asked her, "What did your mother say to you after the doctor told her you were pregnant?" she responded, "She wanted me to leave."

Sociological literature makes two assumptions about Black teenage mothers and their mothers: First, the adult Black mothers are supportive and encourage the daughters to keep and raise the babies. Second, this permissive support is linked to the existence of an extended family support system. In 1974 Carol Stack showed how Black families survive by using extended networks of relatives and friends to help them through tough times. She described "child getting and child keeping" as part of the wonderful and different character of Black family culture.[3] Stack was correct in many of her observations of Black families, but I cannot agree with her assertions about Black families' willingness to let their daughters have and keep their babies.

Supposedly, the chief reason for the mothers' forgiveness is that they have a network of relatives and friends who can offer support.[4] That analysis did not apply to De Vonya and her mother, nor to most of the teen mothers who spoke to me. The major problem with Stack's analysis is that it reduces the complexities of contemporary Black families to the simplicity of a quaint culture in which all Black families

are alike. Such support and extensive kin networks were not com-
monplace among the teen mothers and families I interviewed.

How Black teen mothers and their adult mothers view and handle
their new situation is of theoretical importance given the assumptions
and debates in social science and in the political arena concerning
Black teenage mothers. On one side in this discourse is Patrick Daniel
Moynihan's thesis that Black teenage mothers replicate the values
and attitudes of their mothers. On the other side stands William J.
Wilson, who links the plight of Black mothers to the changes in America's economic structure.[5] But few theories pay sufficient attention to
the impact structural constraints might have on family relationships,
especially between teenage mothers and their mothers. The relationships I observed demonstrate that gender, race, and class inequalities
are reproduced and expressed in the interactions between these Black
teen mothers and their mothers.

Two dominant patterns emerged from these twenty-two interviews:
conflicts between the teen mothers and their mothers grew more intense after the birth of the babies, and the teen mothers defied their
mothers' demands that they have abortions. Before they became
pregnant, most of the teen mothers argued with their mothers over
cleaning their bedrooms, watching television, and doing their homework on time. Some arguments were more intense than others. But
most thought their mothers were generally supportive of them. After
they became pregnant, only ten of the teen mothers found their mothers to be supportive or "somewhat" supportive of them. One of these,
Georgia Minns, a sixteen-year-old, said her mother helped her by
sharing her own experiences as a teen mother. Seventeen-year-old
De Lesha Simons described her mother's attitude this way: "If I knew
that I didn't have my mother standing behind me, I couldn't have had
him." Six of the teen mothers said that their mothers were very angry
at first but became more supportive as time passed. These supportive
mothers were, however, the exceptions.

In contrast, twenty-two of the teen mothers said that their mothers were tremendously angry at them and never forgave them. Fifteen-
year-old Junie Grant's comment was typical: "My mother was not
supportive." Junie angrily declared she was saving her money to
move away from home because of "my relationship with my

momma." The majority of the teen mothers had left or were leaving their mothers' homes because of continual fights over their pregnancies. The older teen mothers still encountered conflict with their mothers, even years after the birth of their babies. Diane Harris, from a middle-class family, thought her mother's feelings about status superseded her love for her daughter: "She looks down on people on AFDC—it's the same thing with teenage mothers." A few teen mothers tried to understand their mother's reaction. Carolyn Mars said of her mother, "I think that she was hurt." Others were more focused on their own needs: "It was like she didn't have any feelings for what my situation might be."

The Deviant Label

The most intense and compelling stories came from teen mothers who said that the least supportive person was their mother. "She called me a bitch and a whore." De Vonya Smalls had a "real battle" with her mother when she heard the news. "Now she doesn't say anything to me. But she could still explode."

Most pregnant teens who had "unsupportive" mothers said those adult mothers responded to the news by assailing their characters. Their mothers' epithets continued throughout the pregnancies, as illustrated by De Vonya's story: "I remember once she was talking to a friend and calling me a whore and a tramp. I heard her in my room talking about me, and I started crying and crying and crying. I left. When I got back, she said, 'You big fat blimp, you don't need to be having this baby. You're too young.' It's like she's never going to forgive me. She told me my baby days are over."

One forty-three-year-old woman, Evie Jenkins, recalled her mother's reaction of twenty-five years before as if it had just happened. With bitterness she remembered, "The bigger I got during my pregnancy, the more my mother hated me. By the time I reached my seventh month, when she came home and she'd look at me, it was like she would close the door to my bedroom. She couldn't stand to look at me. So I finally left." This vignette reveals the longevity of the conflict between nine older women who were previously teen mothers and their mothers. In Evie Jenkins's case, years ago, after the baby's birth, she returned to school to earn a college degree in social work. Despite that accomplishment, her mother continued to imply that she had failed: "My mother has always insinuated that I could have done so much more. But I've ruined my chances for a good marriage and career."

Evie's fight with her mother illustrates the norms and roles associated with the obligations most mothers are expected to fulfill: mothers should always be available and supportive of their children and, given the idealization of motherhood in this society, never waver in that support, regardless of their own problems. The interviews I conducted with these teen mothers illuminate the teens' expectations that nothing in the relationship would change—that norms and values regarding mothering would require their mothers to provide needed support. De Vonya (and most of the teen mothers who thought their mothers unsupportive) expected her mother to mother her again at the same level of support, despite the extra demands an additional child would make on her mother's resources.

The Abortion Issue

All but one of the teen mothers reported that their mothers demanded they have an abortion. The only person whose family said no to an abortion was Lois Patterson, whose grandmother denied her the right to decide: "She told me, 'If you laid down there and had it, you can lay down there and keep it.'" Even mothers who themselves had been teen mothers wanted their daughters to have abortions. For example, Terry Parks, whose mother was emotionally supportive of her, said she had planned on having an abortion because her mother demanded it. Her plans fell through when the baby's father left town without giving her the agreed-upon half of the abortion fee. The teen mother and her mother were hard pressed to come up with the total amount. She said, "Anyway, I'm glad I didn't."

Susan Carter remembered her mother's reaction: "When she found out, my mother said, 'Well, you know you can get an appointment to get an abortion.'" When Cassandra Witt told her mother she was one month pregnant, her mother said she had to agree to have an abortion right away, or she could not live in her house anymore. The teenager was surprised by this strong reaction; until then she and her mother had been fairly close. She moved out that night, stayed at a motel for a few days, and applied for emergency welfare aid. "This is not the life I had in mind," the young mother said.

When asked why they refused to have abortions, De Vonya and most of the teen mothers responded in "us against them" terms. Sixteen-year-old De Vonya said with fervent conviction, "My mother didn't get rid of me." Alicia Cummins, whose baby's father moved to a southern state shortly after she became pregnant, and whose mother pleaded with her to have an abortion, remembered thinking at the time: "I'm going to have my baby, and it's going to be rough but we'll make it." De Vonya's mother called everyone in the family, including the long-absent father, to support her argument that her daughter should have an abortion. When this strategy failed, her mother campaigned for De Vonya to marry the baby's father. The teen mother would not marry a man who refused to acknowledge his baby's existence.

Punishing Strategies

After De Vonya had her baby, she began to think her mother was trying to punish her for not having the abortion: "She dealt with it. But she didn't try to help me or anything. She was givin' me a hard time." Likewise, seventeen-year-old Jasmine Conners, the eldest of five children (and the first of her sisters to become a teenage mother), who lived with her mother and four sisters and brothers in a tiny three-bedroom house in Richmond, related, "She told me, 'You stay in the house. You clean up the kitchen. You do everything. The rest of them can go out. You stay here, in the house, no company, no telephone.' It was like she was punishing me." A year later her fourteen-year-old sister became pregnant.

Was her mother actually punishing her, or was she merely assigning her daughter household tasks as many parents do? Whatever the mother's intentions, her daughter saw the housework assignments as a punitive strategy, and her perception created a great deal of friction between the two of them: "I can't stand her attitude, and she can't stand mine."

De Vonya's mother would not care for any more children. Susan's mother wanted to put her into foster care. "She's thinking about putting me in a foster home and having the baby taken away from me." Susan gave her mother's threats a great deal of thought. If her mother put her away or moved out, as she often warned she might, Susan figured, "If she just left, or put me away, I would run away or I could get a part-time job or something" (her voice rising). Diane Harris told of her mother screaming at her to pack up and move out "immediately." Evie Jenkins, an older teen mother who still remembered her mother closing her bedroom door to avoid seeing her, said that her mother not only refused to acknowledge Evie's pregnancy to anyone who did not have to know but for several years refused to tell anyone she had a grandson.

Some teen mothers felt their status as the baby's primary care giver also challenged by their mother: "You're second banana with your kids," said Melania Lowan. Jackie Marley, another teen mother, complained that her role as mother was undercut by her mother's assumption that she was too immature to be a mother. Jackie concluded her mother was usurping her role and resented her mother for doing so.

Susan Carter provides an example of this general complaint. Susan thought that her mother was being extremely mean to her. According to Susan, her mother continued to treat her like an immature adolescent, taking over the care of her grandchild while, at the same time, complaining that she was "no grandma": "She always makes me feel like I'm not doing a good job. She always puts me down. She told me before that she thinks I should put her up for adoption. My friends tell me I'm doing a good job."

When Evie Jenkins's baby was one year old, she moved into her own apartment. Her mother volunteered to pick up the baby from the baby-sitter and bring him over to Evie's home. "Instead of bringing him home she would just take him over to her house." Conversely, when Evie wanted to go out on the weekends, her mother refused to baby-sit him. Although the teen mother was working part-time and attending night school and thought of herself as a responsible mother, her mother's authority over the grandson went unquestioned:

As a teen mother I was frightened. But I was very responsible for my baby. I mean I went to work when he was two weeks old. But my mother, she almost hit a brick. Because during those times, you couldn't wash your hair for six weeks let alone go to work. The fact that she didn't give me the recognition as a mother affected my relationship with the kid. When I think back, I think what I would have wanted back then was to be taught how to be a mother.

Evie's (and Diane Harris's) wishes for a different response from her mother tell us how much motherhood can impact adolescent girls. Evie wanted her mother to consider her capable. At the same time she wanted further guidance from her mother. This yearning to be both independent of and dependent on her mother speaks to a common adolescent issue that is often misunderstood by their parents and the larger society. Twenty-five years later Evie, who had gone on to college and held a middle-class job, still thought her life was a mess. She was still trying to make sense of her experience as a teenage mother. She had not forgotten her mother's treatment of her nor her experiences on welfare. Evie (and Diane) believed that her life would have been better if she had not gotten pregnant. Perhaps some kind of support system would have helped her move beyond those earlier experiences. She did not receive any help, so she acted on her perception that her life was going down the drain.

Sometimes the teen mothers tried to assert themselves as mothers. Roleta McMann was eighteen and her baby was only a few months old when she moved out of her mother's house. Her mother tracked her down and tried to have the baby taken away from her:

My mother used to call the social worker when I wasn't staying there with her and tell her that I wasn't taking care of my boy right. So my mother took the baby away from me for about eight months. She told my worker that I wasn't feeding him with the money I was getting.

—*Why do you think she called the worker?*

'Cause my mother wanted me to come home and she was trippin' off that. I guess she didn't want me to stay with my auntie. But I knew that's where I wanted to be.

Roleta believed her mother's need to reassert her role as a mother was often satisfied at the expense of Roleta's feelings.

One afternoon I arrived at sixteen-year-old Carmilla Hopkins's home to find the house crowded with relatives. We decided to do the interview at a local restaurant. She assumed that she could take her baby, and she began to dress him. Her mother informed her in a stage whisper that the baby could not go, and she took him away from her. Later that evening, when I asked Carmilla about the incident, she sighed: "I don't ask her to baby-sit when I want to go somewhere unless I want to go somewhere for a short time. Usually she says, 'This is your baby. Stay here and take care of it.' I want to go to a football game and she uses that part about my responsibility to take care of the child. She didn't want me going out. She just wants me staying at home all the time. But I can't do that. I'm still a teenager." As Carmilla recited a list of complaints about her mother, she expressed her ambivalence about her new status. She wanted some flexibility in her roles as both mother and teenager but at the same time expected her mother to be her main source of support.

As illustrated by the teen mothers' quotes above, part of the problem is the question of who should make decisions about the teen mothers' new situation—the teenager or her mother? It was not clear to these mothers who should make decisions—about abortion, marriage, housing, or financial support—or who was responsible for the baby's care. Since it was not apparent to either adult or teen who should make these decisions, the adult mothers often acted in their capacity as authority figures, without discussing the issues with their daughters. De Vonya and other teen mothers wanted their mothers to be more broad-minded and to overcome outdated moral convictions that allowed them to dismiss their daughters' wishes.

Regular Old Ladies

When I asked De Vonya to describe her typical day, she described herself as a "regular old lady." She said her life had become very boring since the baby's birth. "I don't go out with my friends anymore, not even to the movies." Other teen mothers also identified themselves as "a regular old lady." This description was so much a part of their language that when I described one teen mother that way to other teen mothers, they nodded in agreement.

Perhaps the "regular old lady" identifier helped counter the popular view of them as unfit and self-indulgent mothers. I asked the teens if they had fun with their friends anymore. "No!" they said emphatically, since they spent all their spare time with their babies. I told them I found that hard to believe, thinking they were too young to be "old ladies." "No!" they again insisted. I suspect the teen mothers wanted me to see them as good mothers to offset the stereotype of them as dysfunctional teenagers. Of course, their declarations contradicted equally emphatic ones of some, like Carmilla Hopkins, who insisted that while she might be a mother, she was also a teenager.

The Limited Support of the Extended Family

Given that these teen mothers thought their mothers were unsupportive during a crucial time in their lives, I wanted to know who else offered them support during and after their pregnancies. More than three-quarters of them said they counted on one or two friends. Fathers and other kin were absent from the teen mothers' support systems. Only four of the thirty-two mothers said they could rely on other family members for support. Lois Patterson, a twenty-seven-year-old mother who lived with her grandparents and sisters, considered her immediate family and a few friends part of her family support system, but for the most part the help they gave was not consistent, since they had their own money problems. For two teen mothers, it was a matter of pride; as Carolyn Mars explained, "I was just too embarrassed to ask anyone [for help]."

The extended family kinship network certainly played a role in the survival of Black families through the first two-thirds of this century, as Stack correctly notes in her study of Black families. Stack writes about the strength and adaptive strategies used by Black extended families to combat the racism and poverty that left so many without stable jobs. The Black families' kinship networks helped them survive both emotionally and financially. But the Black family structure has greatly changed since Stack published her findings. It may well be, according to Herbert Gutman and Carl N. Degler, that the extended family plays a more important role for southern or midwestern families than for northern or western urban Black families like that of De Vonya Smalls.[6]

The problems are different for rural and urban Black families. For example, urban families, such as those who live in Oakland and Richmond, tend to live farther away from each other than rural families, and their resources are used up faster by higher housing and food costs. Urban families pay higher rent and, as the teen mothers found out when they tried to stay with a friend or relative, have landlords who place restrictions on the number of people who can live in one apartment. In addition, women in urban areas usually work at jobs requiring long hours away from home, and their children are often placed in formal child care systems. Rural women are more likely to work in or close to home or use informal systems like friends or relatives for child care. Living such great distances from relatives who cannot be called on for emotional and financial support and living in inner cities where expenses are high and wages are low, making it impractical to give economic support to others, contributed to the breakdown of the kind of extended families Blacks had in the 1970s as compared with the 1980s, when I interviewed these teen mothers and their mothers.

The typical family pattern of these teen mothers fits the family structure described by Andrew Billingsley as "modified nuclear": one adult in the household raising her own as well as other children. Most of the teenage mothers lived in female-headed households consisting of the mother and children. These families received little if any support from other family members. De Vonya's family of five brothers and sisters, and a father and mother who are each dependent on monthly disability compensation, provides an example of a large Black family with little to offer to what Stack refers to as a mutual exchange system.[7] De Vonya has scant contact with two aunts who live in North Carolina and an uncle who lives in Sacramento. The network that did exist for De Vonya consisted mainly of poor friends who occasionally provided her money for diapers and clothing, transportation to school or day care, and temporary housing. But De Vonya felt that her friends were so often stretched for money or space themselves that she would be an additional burden if she asked for further help.

Moving Day

The one way De Vonya's friends could help her was to let her stay with them until she could make other housing arrangements. Housing arrangements represented a major problem for most of the teen mothers, especially those who wanted to leave their families' homes. The emerging housing problems also crystallized their attitude about their mothers. While twelve teen mothers moved out of their mothers' homes because they needed more space for their new babies, twenty teen mothers, like De Vonya, left home because they could not endure the serious conflicts between them and their mothers. Most of the teen mothers thought they could resolve their problems by leaving their mothers' households. In fact, their problems multiplied—not only did their mothers' attitudes not change, but the teens had to spend a great deal of time finding housing.

It is not clear to me why the housing situation of these young mothers has not been discussed. One visit to the homes of these mothers and their families indicates the need for better housing—especially because most of these teen mothers, like De Vonya, have to live in drug-infested areas. The teen mothers who did live with their mothers, like Susan Carter, usually shared their bedrooms with their babies as well as their sisters. These teen mothers did not have what would be considered a typical teenager's room, filled with records, books, clothes, posters, video games, and school materials. There was almost none of the teenage paraphernalia one might expect to see—just a few teddy bears, plastic toys, games, or baby books. Most of the rooms I saw were tiny and plainly furnished with a twin or double bed and a small dresser. Many of the teen mothers slept with their babies because they could not afford a crib.

Young mothers who are caught up in this lifestyle may actually become transients. One could call them the "nearly homeless": drifting from place to place, staying until they wear out their welcome. Often they feel they are imposing on others. Such unstable arrangements mean that they spend an enormous amount of time devising ways to find housing. Most feel disheartened and upset about their unstable housing arrangements.

The teen mothers' housing situations show the extent to which they could use their fragile support system. Only a few of the older teenage mothers were able to establish stable households. Younger teen mothers, like De Vonya, had to count on a friend or two to lend them sleeping space; sometimes it was on the floor. Some teen mothers moved in with a friend or an "auntie" for a few months, but these arrangements seldom worked. Melania Lowan stayed with a friend for a month until they quarreled over who should clean up after the children. With no other place to go, Melania moved back to her parents' home until the tension there became unbearable again. Then she moved in with her aunt. When I interviewed this seventeen-year-old teen mother, she was in the midst of making new plans: "I want to get out of this apartment by Saturday because the landlord told Deena that her apartment's only big enough for her family. She don't have much room, so I have to move. I can't get housing because I'm too young."

De Vonya, too, had been denied housing because, at sixteen, the landlords said she was too young to apply. For a short time she found housing with friends. De Vonya proudly described how she managed to get around her friend's landlord's occupancy restrictions by sneaking out when the landlord came around to collect the rent. But De Vonya, not being submissive to her situation, did try to find her own apartment and stabilize herself and her daughter's living arrangements. Ultimately, the only apartment of her own that she could find was located in a housing complex considered to be a very dangerous place dominated by a drug organization whose dealers ironically called themselves "the Family." Its leader was famous for hiring bicycle-riding teenage boys to make drug deliveries, paying them more money then they could ever earn at legitimate employment.

The Acorn Housing Complex

De Vonya's new apartment was located in a complex of apartment houses, known as Acorn, developed by private owners and affiliated with the Federal Department of Housing and Urban Development as a subsidized housing site. The housing complex, however, was not under the control of federal agencies; as observers like to say, the complex was under the control of drug dealers.

On our way to De Vonya's new apartment we talked about a *San Francisco Chronicle* newspaper article published several weeks prior to her move reporting that the Oakland police ordered the "gun-toting" security guards at Acorn to give up their shotguns.[8] The tenants had complained about the way housing security guards, hired to discourage the increasing number of drug dealers from carrying on business in the houses, were getting confused about who they were supposed to watch. The tenants reported that the security guards not only set an eleven o'clock curfew for the tenants but applied brutal force against several residents who did not obey the new rules.

I told De Vonya this story as we parked the car in front of her new building. We walked past several smashed cars parked on the street, stepping over the litter of empty beer cans. All of the tenants at Acorn were Black, and approximately 85 percent of the families were headed by "welfare mothers."[9] Acorn's population of single-parent families on welfare reflects the Oakland's Social Services Department's dismal report that "close to 90 percent of female heads of households with children in Oakland live in poverty and receive AFDC assistance."

On our way into De Vonya's apartment building, we passed a group of teenagers who were listening to a loud rap song on a black, sleek "ghetto blaster." Several boys, African chains dangling against their shirts, swayed with the music. We walked up the three flights to De Vonya's one-bedroom apartment and opened the door to be greeted by a strong smell of paint. Dirty worn linoleum squeaked beneath our feet. De Vonya seemed pleased to be moving into the apartment; she smiled as we investigated the closets and bathroom.

We laughingly called the apartment the "penthouse," because it was the only one located on the third (and last) floor. From the "penthouse" bedroom windows we looked down on broken liquor bottles littering the roof of the building next door. De Vonya thought the building's cleaning people had left the garbage there. I told her I thought the garbage on the roof meant those drug dealers were using the roof. "Whatever! I can't worry about that now!" she snapped. When we returned to the car to pick up more boxes, a tough-looking man approached me mumbling words I could not understand. De Vonya whispered, "He's dealin' drugs and wants to sell you some."

Several days later, as we sat together on the bare floor in De Vonya's living room planning where to place imaginary furniture, she suggested we take a walk. I jumped at the suggestion, since the apartment was becoming uncomfortably warm. We walked across the street to a small park to sit between two shady oak trees. Suddenly, the loud whirring noise of a police helicopter's rotors overhead interrupted our conversation. "Surely it will go away," I said. She seemed to take the noise in stride as she informed me that the police may have been keeping us under surveillance as possible drug dealers. I laughed at the vision of me being handcuffed and hauled into the police station as a suspect. De Vonya, alert and healthy, did not seem to be involved in drugs; nor did little La Shetta, who lay contentedly in her stroller, show signs of malnutrition or other problems associated with a mother's drug abuse. We tried to continue our discussion, but the helicopter stayed, too. After a while we gave up and left the park.

Several days after the interview with De Vonya, when I expressed concern over the teen mothers' unstable and unsuitable housing arrangements, a staff member at the Alternative Center pulled out one of their pamphlets: "One of the major problems facing the [Center] now is finding housing for Oakland's homeless pregnant adolescents and teen mothers." The counselors worried that the teen mothers' efforts to find housing would undermine the strides they were making in turning their lives around.

The teen mothers sought new housing in order to change their relationships with their mothers. The teen mothers perceived their mothers' refusal of support as a repudiation of their obligation as mothers rather than as evidence of their mothers' powerlessness. De Vonya and the other teen mothers wanted their mothers to have a progressive moral authority that would overcome outdated moral convictions that led them to reject their daughters. Those moral convictions legitimize the wider society's view that mothering is women's essential nature. The adult mothers had a difficult time living up to those assumptions and so further alienated the teenage girls, who were already feeling alienated and isolated, and worsened their relationships.

As we might expect, and as we will see in the next chapter, the mothers of these teen mothers, including De Vonya's, had their own views of their daughters' situations and their abilities to change their lives.

Part Two

The Family's Response

Chapter Four

The Adult Mothers

It's not my fault, so why do I have to be blamed for what happened to her?

Jennie Shimms, mother of a teenage mother

Early one morning as I arrived at Susan Carter's house for our scheduled interview, I was greeted by her mother, Janet, who informed me that Susan was not awake yet. Since Susan was not awake, this seemed a good time to talk with her mother about her own feelings concerning Susan's situation. Janet Carter, a tall, thin woman, dressed for work in a fashionable black corduroy ankle-length dress, closely resembled her attractive daughter. Stabbing the air with outstretched fingers, Janet expressed how furious she was with Susan for causing her so many problems—all of which she attributed to Susan's "irresponsible nature." Her fingers counted out her daughter's many misdeeds: "She stays out late and leaves the baby with me more than she should. She refuses to do any housework and sleeps late every day." Janet did not feel ready to be a grandmother, and she added "Dammit" to emphasize the point.

The Mothering Obligation

In this society's view women, not men, are charged with caring for others and for the moral training of their children. Caring for others and teaching them social values are the hallmarks of women's mothering obligations and an important basis for what Nancy Russo calls

67

the motherhood mandate, which includes the obligation to be a good mother.[1] This theory of the family directly connects the family structure to patriarchy: fathers provide the economic leadership and authority, and mothers are responsible for the reproduction of children's mainstream values and behavior. Especially during the early and teenage years, the mother's role in social reproduction is considered crucial.

According to this motherhood mandate, all women are expected to mother their children. Some studies argue, however, that Black mothers who are single, as opposed to Black mothers in two-parent households or White mothers in general, have a distinctive set of beliefs, values, and behavior patterns that tend to perpetuate their own socioeconomic conditions. Such studies conclude that women in Black female-headed families produce more of their kind: teenage girls with few values who become teenage mothers, serving as an affront to the values and norms of the general society.[2]

What is significant in this study is the meanings these adult mothers make of their daughters' situations in concert with the daughters' perspectives of their mothers.[3] Adding tremendous weight to these meanings are the influences of the adult mothers' economic status. Four of ten adult mothers interviewed for this study were poor, earning an average income of $6,000 to $8,000; two working-class mothers earned yearly incomes of $11,000 to $13,000; and four were middle-class professionals with a yearly income of $25,000 to $45,000.

All of the adult mothers were deeply disappointed with their daughters. When Virginia Blake's daughter told her she was pregnant, Virginia, who also had a younger child, knew she could not support another one. She said she was alarmed, angry, and resentful. Carmilla Hopkins's mother, who needed support from AFDC for herself and her younger child, confessed it was a most upsetting and difficult time for her. Janet Carter confided that it was hard for her to admit that all of her lectures to Susan on not becoming sexually involved with boys before she was an adult did nothing to stop her daughter from becoming sexually active. Janet's observations could also be applied to those neighborhood "old women" whose gossip and negative sanctioning of teenage girls did not stop the increase of teenage pregnancies.

The adult mothers were more difficult to interview than the teen mothers. Most were either too busy or too tired to sit through the interviews. Nonetheless, this was an important group to consider because their views are not usually reflected in literature on Black mothers.

These adult mothers' interviews do not support the popular view that teenage pregnancies and motherhood are condoned by Black families and the Black community, which is based on the idea that the Black and White cultures hold extremely different values for their children. Rather, they confirm a central theme of this book: teenage pregnancies break several important and long-standing cultural norms greatly valued by adult Black mothers.

Interestingly, although the adult mothers came from poor, working-class, and middle-class backgrounds, neither class variation nor the adult mothers' status as former teen mothers made a difference to the problems they had with their teenage daughters. But class variations and the adult mothers' status as teen mothers impacted the *meaning* they made of their daughters' pregnancies. These social factors were also useful in creating two categories of adult mothers: the class aspirers and the class sliders.[4]

The concepts refer to the adult mothers' aspirations regarding their dreams, desires, abilities, and place within the economic structure. The adult mothers sought to fulfill those desires through their daughters. Lower-income mothers, who I refer to as class aspirers, felt their pregnant teenage daughters had failed them. Until their daughters' pregnancies, this group had hoped their daughters would do better with their lives than they had and through educational achievement attain a higher class status. The mothers hoped their daughter's success would trickle down to them. The mothers I refer to as class sliders had come from humble beginnings and had worked hard to achieve and preserve their image of middle-class respectability. These middle-class mothers felt cheated when their daughters became pregnant. They tended to believe that teenage pregnancy reflected the kind of sexual behavior associated with the lower classes.

Poor and Working-Class Adult Mothers: Class Aspirers

Notions of upward mobility echoed throughout these interviews. These adult mothers stressed their aspirations for their daughters to lead the good life, climb the class ladder, and help the family do so as well. Adult mothers with low incomes like Janet Carter, who had such high hopes for their daughters, took their daughters' pregnancies quite hard. Sometimes the adult mothers tried to put their views across by putting themselves down. Sadly, the class aspirers felt that the only way to handle their own experiences as teenage mothers was to serve as a negative role model for their daughters— of "what not to do," as Etta Marley told me.

Janet and Susan Carter

Janet Carter could not depend on Joney, the baby's father, to help her support her grandchild: he was serving a two-year sentence in a correctional facility for delinquent adolescents. His mother sent the baby an occasional gift of clothing and Pampers, but it was not substantial. With an additional person to feed and care for because, Janet Carter thought, her daughter was not a good mother, she felt stuck: "Susan should give up the baby to foster care, to someone who can take care of it. Maybe you can talk some sense into her." The tone of her voice made the frustrated woman's words seem like a veiled threat to take some action against her daughter. After a few minutes of listening to Janet, I began to sense that she was mainly interested in dispelling any ideas I may have had about linking her to her daughter's moral behavior, that perhaps she spoke of putting her grandchild into foster care to say these problems were her daughter's own fault, not related to Janet's failure as a parent. It was Susan's mother, Janet, and not the baby's father, who would be blamed for failing to socialize her daughter to conform to gender- and age-appropriate behavior regarding sexual behavior and early childbearing. In other words, Janet viewed herself, not Susan, as the real victim. She was obviously under great stress, both financial and emotional. Her shoulder slumped a little as she headed for the door to go to work. As she closed the door, it was clear my reassurances to her were vapid and Pollyannaish.

As the interviews illustrate, Susan's mother was not the only one to react with frustration and anger at the news of her daughter's pregnancy. The small sample of ten adult mothers in this study certainly illuminated the feminists' view of the way mothers are held accountable for their daughters' sexual behavior. Awareness of this accountability may have been a factor in the decision of over half the adult mothers to refuse to take part in this study, and it may have contributed to the dynamics between them and their daughters when I visited. In some cases, if the mothers were at home when I interviewed their daughters, they scarcely acknowledged my presence. A few interrupted the interviews when they had something to say to their daughters. Some banged pots and pans as they went about cooking dinner, so that the teen mother and I could hardly communicate.

Unlike Janet Carter, Mary Smalls had been a teenage mother herself. (Thirteen of the adult mothers of the thirty-two teenage mothers had been teenage mothers.) The two mothers were different in other ways as well. Mary was older than Janet, earned less money, and was beset by health problems. But there was a striking similarity. Both mothers received little support from other family members. Mary did not have a man present, or anyone else, for that matter, to help her with the children. Janet's mother, seventy-six years old and in good health, was available to help out. But the grandmother—who issued orders, advice, and criticism about her daughter's and granddaughter's lives—did not feel she had to help Janet with the children.[5]

Mary and De Vonya Smalls

Mary Smalls, a thin and slightly stooped woman, took time away from ironing clothes late one afternoon to describe how hard work and worry had broken her health, her stamina, and her spirit, forcing her to stop working: "I would stand on my feet and stuff and I would work twelve hours a day. And my muscles and things in my back would start to hurt. . . . It got to the place where I couldn't even stand for the clothes to touch my back. It would hurt me." Mary reminisced about getting married at sixteen, six months before the birth of her first child. "In those days we had what we called shotgun weddings." Her husband, Mary found out later, was a "fall-down drunk," who she picked up from the floor so often that she permanently injured her back. He was remembered mainly for his audacity to leave the family two days after De Vonya's birth.

In most ways Mary's story was one of survival. As Patricia Hill
Collins writes about Black mothers, "Affection must often wait until
the basic needs of physical survival are satisfied."[6] Mary had main-
tained a stable home for six children, although in many months the
rent check bounced. She always managed to talk the landlord into
holding off the eviction notice for a few weeks. Despite this testa-
ment to her capacities, Mary Smalls saw her life as "pure drudgery."
Her life seemed even more difficult when she watched two other
daughters work at a series of dead-end jobs and then marry "a couple
of deadbeats," who left them with children, forcing them to get on
welfare.

Mary's comments point to the way the emotional elements shaped
these adult mothers' perceptions of the limited roles they play in their
daughters' lives. In describing her lack of influence, Mary said she felt
even more frustrated and discouraged with De Vonya, her youngest
child: "I wanted her to go to college because this is what she keeps
talking about. I didn't want De Vonya to work in White people's
homes. I was hurt when she got pregnant before she had finished
school and could graduate, and now she be like me." Now Mary has
been cheated out of watching her daughter go to college.

When De Vonya told her mother that the school counselors wanted
her to go to an alternative school, Mary became quite angry with her
daughter for causing her even more problems. Several months later,
she was more resigned. "That's life," she sighed, her small voice con-
veying the sentiment of other Black mothers with "one more cross to
bear."[7]

In talking about her life, Mary matched her experiences with those
of her daughter. She had vivid memories of being isolated as a teenage
mother from her friends. She remembered the cruel gossip and her
mother's sharp tongue when she called Mary a "whore," while at the
same time demanding that she marry the baby's father, "drunk or not."
The memories, still fresh in her mind, helped her empathize with her
daughter. Still, she would not let her daughter fail again, she told me.
"No second chance" was the major lesson Mary wanted De Vonya to
learn: "Okay, my daughter made a mistake. She's human. It was just
that heat of the moment. But I say to myself there ain't no way she's
going to stay on welfare and have a bunch of babies."

Joyce Ladner notes that mothers who have also been teenage mothers strongly desire their daughters to lead a different kind of life. "The notion of do as I say not as I do was pervasive. . . ."[8] Denise Collins's mother, who had her first child at sixteen, feared that everyone would think she was a failure as a mother. Supposedly she lacked the ability to socialize Denise correctly, lost parental control over her, and passed on her own low moral standards to her daughter.

Mary Smalls believed she had raised her daughter well, and she wanted to reinforce the idea that she would not tolerate a second mistake; she would do this by making sure De Vonya take full responsibility for her child. "This is my daughter's responsibility," she said a little sharply. Perhaps perceiving how I might interpret her tone of voice, she suddenly smiled, softening her voice: "It's not like I'm trying to punish her, but I have to remind her of her mistake."

The edge returned to Mary's voice: "I wanted to be a good grandmother. But I'm tired and have health problems. See, I have migraine headaches and I'm not suppose to get upset too much. 'Cause the last test I had, it seems like I've got a nerve in my head that kicks off every once in a while. And I have seizures so I can't deal with these problems too much."

The adult and teen mothers frequently complained about their health problems. Several of the adult mothers were badly overweight and suffered from hypertension. Seventeen of the teen mothers reported stress-related problems: car accidents and job-related accidents. De Vonya had had two breast cancer operations. Evie Jenkins had had two heart attacks. Another teen mother was suffering from back problems. When I mentioned these health problems to the counselors at the Alternative Center, they told me they had compiled their own reports of such women's health care problems. Their findings support a number of others indicating that a high percentage of Black women with low income suffer from "higher incidences of stressful life events and higher rates of psychological disorder than many others."[9] Low-income Black women also report more cases of hypertension and diabetes than other groups of women. Another study notes that the majority of these mothers, women in their thirties, experience severe hardships. Black female-headed households experience more acute stress and have fewer people in their support groups than White families.

Middle-Class Status Sliders

A recurring theme in the stories of the middle-class teen mothers like Evie Jenkins and Diane Harris was their upward mobilization as teenagers whose loving family relationships deteriorated during their pregnancies. The mothers of Evie Jenkins and Diane Harris fit the model of middle-class mothers who worry that their prestige and status in the community have been threatened by their teenage daughters' pregnancies. In Goffman's view, the adult mothers saw their daughters' pregnancies as a sign that their families had "slipped": "I refer to the adult mothers in this group as 'class sliders.'" Goffman would say that the adult mothers' reactions were a defensive measure against the "soiled" identity of their daughters. The "assumption being that [she] is what the others are."[10] These adult mothers believed that becoming a teen mother was lower-class behavior and that their daughter's pregnancy was a step down the class prestige ladder—which they had struggled so hard to climb up.

The stress these adult mothers felt was evident. Several middle-class adult mothers were concerned about losing their jobs because of the school board's ongoing threats of cutbacks. One middle-class adult mother, Marie Jenkins, felt stressed, complaining of frequent headaches and colds.

Evie and Marie Jenkins

Whereas sixteen-year-old De Vonya's and her mother's lives seemed like one struggle after another, forty-three-year-old Evie Jenkins recalled her early teenage years as being fairly stable and middle-class. Evie, a tall, stout woman, opened the door of her apartment in a Richmond housing complex and led me into a modest-sized living room filled with traditional furniture, plants, and a Steinway piano. A congenial woman, she seemed to laugh easily, yet she cried when she talked about her own "unsupportive" mother. She made faces when she talked about her experiences with the welfare program. When we met, she was recovering from a second heart attack and had needed to apply for disability insurance.

Given that she started out with more advantages because of her family's background, life should have worked out better for Evie Jenkins than for De Vonya Smalls. Evie's mother, Marie, the first in her family to hold a teaching degree, taught in the San Francisco school district until she retired a few years before. Evie's father was a cook for Amtrak. Evie's parents worked hard to elevate themselves to a middleclass lifestyle. They expected Evie to continue their own educational tradition; she would go to college and become a doctor or perhaps follow in her mother's footsteps as a teacher. Her mother said of Evie: "I wanted her to really be something, to go on and finish school, and I wanted to send her to Europe, to just be something other than a mother." Instead, Evie became pregnant at seventeen, dropped out of high school, and, a few months later, became a welfare mother. She spent the next ten years on welfare. Toward the end of those years, she decided she could not stay on welfare forever and celebrated her ninth year on AFDC by enrolling in a college course. Several years later she was celebrating again after earning her degree in social work. In the next two years her life changed drastically: she married Charlie, the baby's father, had another child, divorced Charlie, and found a job as a caseworker for the welfare administration. "It's ironic," she said with a laugh, "There I was, working for the same agency that had given me money and a hard time, now hiring me to give others money and a hard time."

Evie was proud of turning her life around. She remembered the years she spent as a teenage mother as the most painful time of her life. The interviews helped clarify one troubling issue for her: with all the work she put into redirecting her life, she realized she never regained her mother's faith in her. "My mother will always think of me as a failed woman."

Evie Jenkins's mother, Marie, an articulate and handsome woman of seventy-three, said of her daughter's pregnancy of years before, "It was a stigma." Her daughter's behavior had infuriated the stately woman, who lived by strict rules: "I taught Evie to listen to me and to be careful of her reputation." Marie's reaction to her daughter's pregnancy is not hard to understand; after all, like most of the other middle-class adult mothers, she had worked hard most of her life to attain some measure of respect and prestige and had had moderate success with the climb up the class ladder. Marie voiced those concerns by saying, "It's just disappointing to me the way she turned out.

Maybe I expected too much for her. She's been on welfare for a long time. All those wasted years. She'll never catch up. I have tried to instill in her a sense of pride, but she doesn't pay me any attention."

Evie remembered feeling that as the first in her family to become a teenage mother and to apply for welfare, she had committed two wrongs:

My mother hated me for it. I was just alone. I just felt alone (voice trembles). You have to excuse me (sobbing). It brings back a lot of horrible memories. It had to do with the pregnancy. And she didn't tell anybody she had a grandchild until he was three years old. My mother was educated and had a job. My father had a job. So therefore they took care of everything. The only problem I had was that my mother did not stand me. She just couldn't stand to look at me. I had to go stay on my own for a while.

Evie closed her eyes and pushed herself further into the armchair's cushions.

The bigger I got during my pregnancy, the more my mother hated me. She bought everything for the baby. She bought me maternity clothes. But by the time I reached my seventh month, she couldn't stand to look at me.

Evie moved out of her home for a few months. She stayed at a friend's house and then moved back home: "We quarreled constantly." She moved again several months later; on reflection she wished she had moved earlier. She also remembered her mother's letting her know that the neighbors were gossiping about her: "She told me I was being called names. I was called a whore. I was labeled *bad* [emphasizes word], an evil influence. She just left me completely alone to face these names."

Now, twenty-five years later, she acknowledged that she was still unable to mend the relationship with her mother. Evie's mother's inability to "forgive" her daughter demonstrates the ferocity of the stigma of teenage pregnancy. The grandmother did not, as her daughter had hoped, get over her anger and step in to take care of her daughter and grandchild. Such longevity and intensity characterized these daughter-mother relationships. Evie was also astonished by the animosity in her own voice: "She'll never forgive me, and I ain't gonna forgive her."

What is most compelling in Evie's and other teen mother's stories is that all of them seemed to find their experiences as teen mothers so debilitating and disabling that they lived them over and over again—an indication that they had not recovered from those ordeals despite the moderate success they achieved later in life.[11]

Alma and Diane Harris

Diane Harris and her mother Alma's relationship varied in detail, but in general it was quite similar to Evie's and Marie's. Diane Harris's mother wanted to make up with her daughter. Alma, a local elementary school teacher, believed that only girls with "ghettoized mentality," living in the kind of inner-city cultural environment where teenage pregnancy was a way of life, became pregnant. How did she explain her daughter's pregnancy at seventeen? Impeccably dressed, Alma Harris sat on the edge of her dining room chair and filled our coffee cups as she answered: "Well, obviously she met a ghetto-type jerk who managed to convince her to do what he wanted. He doesn't have much of a future. He's only a high school graduate who works part-time at a construction firm. He was not the kind of man I had in mind for my daughter."

Alma's family had come a long way from their two-bedroom apartment in an old, run-down apartment building in West Oakland near the glitzy Paramount Theater. When Diane's father landed a job at an Oakland engineering firm, they used the savings they had diligently put aside each month to buy a spacious house in the Oakland hills with a view of San Francisco.

Diane's paternal grandmother Louise often visited their home, walking up the steep hill from the bus stop on unsteady feet, strands of gray hair peeking out from a red wig perched carelessly on her head. She usually arrived at the Harris's home loudly cursing anyone who managed to get in her way. Alma viewed Louise with shame and suspicion. She was the only reminder of the family's past, and she served as a reminder that the family should keep check on their manners and behavior so that neighbors would not mistake them for "ghetto types." Ignored was the fact that Louise raised her only child (Alma's husband and Diane's father) singlehandedly by cleaning office buildings in downtown Oakland during the night shift.

When Diane recalled a distant cousin on her father's side who received AFDC for a year when she lost her job, Alma Harris let it be known that she did not know her husband's cousin that well. Diane explained, "My mother doesn't know people on AFDC, or teenage mothers." Diane, a pretty, diminutive twenty-year-old who fancied tank tops, cut-away jeans, and gold earrings, could not forgive her mother for treating her so badly when she was pregnant. Diane responded to my question, "Who is the least supportive person?" with a shrug of her shoulders: "My mother and her family." She recounted the ugly scene the night she told her mother she was pregnant. They quarreled until two in the morning, when Alma told Diane to have an abortion: "I said, 'No!' Well, she told me, 'If you're not going to have an abortion, get out!' " At first Diane did not believe her mother, but when her mother stopped talking to her, it became apparent she meant it. Diane grabbed pieces of clothing, stuffed them into a suitcase, and took a taxi cab to a friend's house. Alma recalled it differently: "She just left, just walked out when I told her I thought she should have an abortion. I think I was hurt. . . . She didn't care about the family's reputation."

In trying to understand her mother's reaction, Diane thought her mother's fear of gossiping neighbors may have gotten in the way of her feelings about her daughter. Although Diane disagreed with her mother about the abortion and whether she should stay at home, she fundamentally shared her mother's shame and fear of losing status. Class difference was important to her.

Using her middle-class status as a wedge between herself and the other teen mothers, Diane stressed again and again that she was not like those "lower-class girls" who had babies because they grew up in a "casual" culture. "What makes you different?" I asked. Her pregnancy was simply an accident, she said: "They have kids—that's the thing to do, their moral character being flaky. My pregnancy was an accident." Like Evie, Diane remained resentful of her mother. But this time it was the daughter who did not forgive the mother.

Joanne and Selma Wright

Class issues came up again in an interview with Joanne Wright, a thirty-five-year-old reentry law student from a middle-class family, who also became estranged from her mother, Selma, during her pregnancy. Joanne recalled how much her mother resented her and how gossip hurt: "My memory of my childhood was that I was happy until I was fifteen, then the shit hit the fan." Her mother, a social worker and a deaconess at her church, carried herself as a model of moral virtue. She was held in high regard by the church and the community, and she wanted her daughter to emulate her.

Joanne was short, slender, and not shy about wearing bright lipstick. With her trace of southern accent she described an explicit set of complex rules regarding the obligation of mothers, only hinted at in Diane's and Evie's interviews. Daughters were expected to exhibit the same moral values as their mothers: "My mother's sense of morals had to do with my pregnancy at an early age and my being unmarried. My sense of morals came from my mother. I wanted to be married and to not have a baby at an early age." Indeed, she did share many of her mother's moral beliefs about conformity to gender- and age-appropriate behavior: "[The gossiping neighbors] made my mother feel as if she had failed [as an example of moral leadership in the community] because of me. . . . My mother thought she had failed. She, as well as me, were being talked about. And that was the first sign in my family that all was not well." Joanne's mother saw her family disgraced by the ugly rumors surfacing about her daughter. As Joanne viewed it, her mother grew increasingly concerned with the gossip about them and the need to separate herself from her daughter: "My mother could not overcome her moral sense, and this had a tremendous impact on our relationship—it created a gap between us."

Joanne's mother demanded that her daughter make a public confession of her "sins" to her church's congregation, asking for forgiveness. Joanne did as Selma Wright demanded; she remembered the day she stood up in church and asked for forgiveness. But she was furious at her mother for embarrassing her in front of the entire congregation, some of whom were classmates she had known all of her life. She moved out of her mother's home a few months later.

Joanne's mother found it far more difficult than the church to forgive her daughter for damaging her public image. When Joanne recently told her mother she had just registered for college, her mother informed her, in an exasperated tone, that she doubted Joanne could do anything well.

Impression Management Strategies

Besides their concern over their friends and neighbors' negative perception of them as mothers, the class sliders and the class aspirers had something else in common. They used similar "covering" strategies to deal with the stigma of having a teenage mother as a daughter. Even now, all of Joanne's mother's friends believe her daughter to be three years older than her actual age. Evie's mother closed her daughter's bedroom and refused to see her grandson for several years. Other adult mothers went to greater lengths to control information on their daughters. According to counselors at the Alternative Center, it is not unusual for middle-class Black families to put their daughters in homes (like the Florence Crittenton Center for Girls in San Francisco). Virginia Blake and her mother persuaded her fifteen-year-old daughter, Annie, that she should stay at a home for delinquent girls until the baby was born. That experience was indelibly stamped on Annie Blake's mind:

There was a gate. That's what I didn't like. I remember my mother and grandmother taking me up there, and I saw this big iron gate on the door. And I said, "Oh God, this is a prison I'm at and I'm stuck here." I was mad because I didn't want to go. But my mom kept saying, "It's better for you." It was really dirty. The pipes broke in the bathroom, and the water ran all over the place. And they had dirty, stinky carpets in all the rooms.

I was upset. [My family's] main concern was putting the baby up for adoption. They said that nobody will know. And I said, "It's my choice to go or not." And they weren't supportive at all, although they did let me come home after a while when I screamed at them and got so sick they had to take me out.

Annie Blake went home to her mother and grandmother and kept her baby, as well as her anger at her family.

Another strategy adult mothers used is one I call "redirecting the gaze." Some mothers, like Susan's and Diane's, criticized their daughters during the interviews as if they were trying to shift the focus away from themselves. Janet's fear that her reputation would be besmirched by her daughter's may have prompted her to stress over and over that she had tried hard to raise her daughter well, that her daughter's pregnancy was not a reflection of her capability as a mother but rather of her lack of influence over her daughter and her daughter's own nature: "What can you do, when she wants to hang out all day with those characters from school. She's just like them." The adult mothers were caught in a dilemma. If Janet Carter offered Susan support, others might pass on the stigma of her daughter's deviant status to her. These adult mothers may see their daughters' situation as a sign that "these girls have no guidance," a judgment of their own maternal abilities and moral codes.

Cultural Norms

Why did these adult mothers react so negatively to their daughters? According to Frank Furstenberg Jr., the mother who has nurtured and guided the child in her early years may punish the teenager she sees as immoral, especially when feeling challenged by the teenager, whom she considers to be under her authority. When the new baby is born, old ideas about the proper age at which parenthood should be achieved may become manifest. It should not be surprising then to find Susan's, Diane's, or Joanne's mother clinging to "ideas about rigid age and gender expectation."[12] These powerful gender expectations also figured in shaping these adult mothers' reactions to their daughters.

The adult mothers were reacting to the breaking of at least three strongly held gender expectations, or norms, about childbearing and sexuality. The first concerns the age and manner in which women should have children. Young women should certainly not have children until they reach adult status, and not before marriage. What we see in most cases is an unspoken, but mutually agreed, acceptance of these norms about age, motherhood, and marriage. For example, when these adult mothers were children, they were taught to obey those moral rules about girls' sexual behavior. Most said they gave their daughters the same message they had received from their mothers: "good girls" did not have sex, and bad girls did. Janet Carter, remembering her own mother's warning, cautioned her daughter: "You better not even discuss sex, let alone have it, with anyone until you get yourself married and talk about it to your husband. No man wants to marry soiled goods."

The second moral norm—that sexually active unmarried girls become "soiled goods"—follows from the first. Janet Carter said she found it quite a blow to her reputation when she had to acknowledge to friends that her daughter, barely into her adolescence, was sexually active. Now everyone in Janet's circle of friends knew her daughter's sexual history. Implicit in this statement is a notion Edwin Schur captures best: "Only poor, ignorant, and mentally ill girls" become pregnant at an early age. "Nice girls don't."[13]

The third social norm that aggravated the relationship between daughters and mothers was the notion that successful mothering means passing on social values to children. Like many of the other adult mothers, Janet took her daughter's pregnancy as a sign of her own inability to influence her daughter. She did not know what to do when Susan became pregnant. She had no strategy in place to handle her anger when she finally forced the "awful news" from Susan. "I didn't have control over her. So I resorted to calling her names, because I didn't know what else to do."

The third social norm, as exposed in Janet's feelings of losing control over her daughter, underscores a crucial element of the motherhood mandate: mothers should be able to exert control over their daughters' sexual behavior. Therefore, when a teenage daughter becomes pregnant, the norms about her mother's (but not her father's) ability to socialize the daughter gain in significance. Mothers have to be concerned that their daughter's failure may be linked to them. If the adult mother has been a teen mother herself, like Mary Smalls, she fears that her daughter's failure will be perceived as her own moral failure. If she is middle-class, like Alma Harris, she may feel others will think she did not have the ability to control her daughter. Bearing out these fears, the teen mothers were filled with stories of their mothers' concerns that friends were gossiping about them, reflecting the cultural taboo against "age-inappropriate" sexual behavior.

Susan Carter's and Joanna Wright's mothers certainly believed that their family, friends, neighbors, and even fellow church members held them accountable for their daughters' moral values and therefore their sexual activities and pregnancies.

Gender and Economics in the Experience of Black Mothers

When Janet Carter left Susan and her sisters home, unsupervised and bored, while she worked, she did so only because she could not afford to pay for after-school care: "The cheapest rate I found for one child was eighty dollars a week, and for two children they give you a reduction. But it's still ridiculous." She described stepping out her door each morning on her way to work only to see the drug dealers and other signs of urban blight. Some mornings, when Janet's money had run out, she found herself searching through dresser drawers and digging in the children's pockets for small change. Inside the crowded apartment, she showed me how she made space for her grandchild's crib by pushing Susan's bed and dresser together. She was not a lazy and ignorant mother raising an irresponsible, lazy, and ignorant daughter. She was hardworking and aspiring, and she wanted Susan to excel, to move beyond the levels of poverty and stress she had to endure. For poor mothers (Mary Smalls, for example) or working mothers (like Janet Carter), poverty is ongoing; for middle-class mothers (like Alma Harris), memories of childhood poverty and the fear that poverty might be just over the horizon if they lose their jobs—a very likely possibility—drive them to censure their daughters.[14]

The burden on the adult mothers in this study is evident in their emotional reactions to their daughters. Mary Smalls was defensive. It was her daughter's fault, she said, and she felt trapped by the added responsibilities. The chance that the poorly educated woman could simply walk away was slim, if at all possible, she believed. She had less freedom and right than her husband to "chuck it all." She was the one who had to stay for the children, Mary Smalls reminded me, rushing through a list of rhetorical questions: "My husband, he leaves. Where would I find the money to leave? Where would I go? How would I live?"

Mary's reference to gender differences in her comparison between her husband's life and her own is supported by sociologist Maxine Baca Zinn's argument: "The problems of male joblessness and female-headed households form themselves around gender. Although these conditions are the result of economic transformations, they change gender relations as they change the marital, family and labor arrangements of women and men."[15] Baca Zinn's assumptions, coupled with the emotional burden of single adult mothers having conventional mainstream values, hit home when I heard Mary Smalls, described by De Vonya as being overburdened and emotionally withdrawn, refuse to help her daughter.

The adult Black mothers in this study seemed to be overtaxed and overextended by the demands of their daughters' situations. The grandmothers in a study by Joyce Ladner complained about their own unmet emotional and social needs and feelings of being "powerless" to cope with their children's demands. They reported that their children showed them no respect, did not listen to their advice, and placed little value on their role as parents. Ladner also writes that these mothers "did not welcome the [daughter's] pregnancy." [16]

Mary Smalls responded to her feelings that both De Vonya's and her own life were getting out of control by becoming the stern "task master." She pushed De Vonya to find her own housing. Perhaps that push was her way of making her daughter more responsible and less like her irresponsible father. De Vonya did not see it that way. De Vonya, a very perceptive sixteen-year-old, made her analysis very clear to me. Once, for a fleeting moment, De Vonya quietly and hesitantly acknowledged the tremendous price her mother paid for doing everything without getting any support for herself: "I guess from me being the youngest and the pressure she went through with the other ones . . . she's probably burned out."

De Vonya believed that her mother had grown so weary of day-to-day struggles that she had lost the capacity to love her youngest daughter. Despite this understanding of her mother, De Vonya also revealed a presumption for herself that speaks for all of these teen mothers: no matter how much she comprehended her mother's situation, she still expected to be mothered: "My mother's tired of me, and I'm tired of her attitudes too." If her mother loved her, the teenage mother asked in a baffled voice, "Wouldn't she have been more understanding? After all, it happened to her, too."

De Vonya's expectation about her mother's responsibility was in accord with those regarding all women in our society, regardless of class and race: mothers are expected to care for their children. These mothers' notions about motherhood fit with the idea that while the Black community is liberal on political issues, it tends to be conservative on moral and religious issues.[17] But a closer look reveals that in Black households "child keeping," as Stack puts it, exacts a heavy toll from both the teen mothers and their adult mothers.[18] I heard the strain in Mary Smalls's voice. I also heard the anxiety in Alma Harris's voice, a woman so driven to guard her middle-class status that she turned away from her daughter.

I suspect that the teenage daughters' need for further mothering— to be daughters again—cannot be satisfied by their adult mothers.[19] Adult mothers cannot afford to keep mothering their teenage daughters, economically, socially, or emotionally. But these daughters saw their mothers from the perspective of angry, frustrated, and confused adolescence, and without an understanding of the socioeconomic problems that forced their mothers to take such a strong stance. If Janet Carter, Mary Smalls, and Alma Harris viewed their situation as one in which they had been shortchanged by their daughters, they did so out of fear that as single mothers they had to take on most of the economic and emotional responsibilities for their daughters and grandchildren. If, as Moynihan and others claim, these women failed as mothers, it is because they, like their daughters, had no resources and were basically alone. They lacked a steady income and an extended family network to do the kind of mothering required by the motherhood mandate.

Chapter Five

The Babies' Fathers

He left and I just felt basically alone.

Seventeen-year-old Melania Lowan

At the same time De Vonya Smalls, Susan Carter, and the other teen mothers were confronting increasing challenges with their mothers, their relationships with the babies' fathers were also changing. Only two teen mothers mentioned having supportive men. One of them, Carolyn Mars, said, "When I decided to keep the baby, he couldn't have been happier." Another four teen mothers reported that their babies' fathers visited them and the babies once or twice a month. Still, these teen mothers also reported that their lives were difficult. In the two cases with supportive men, the teen fathers were unemployed and depended on the teen mothers' welfare checks.

The remaining twenty-six teen mothers knew very little about their babies' fathers' personal histories or their current lives. What they did say revealed a deeply complex and troubling portrait of young Black men as fathers. This portrait of fathers came mostly from the teen mothers' perspectives and my own observations; literature on men and fatherhood filled in the rest of the picture.

Most teen fathers were between seventeen and twenty years old when their babies were born. In most cases there was a two- to three-year age difference between the teen mother and the teen father. When she became pregnant, Junie Grant was fourteen and her baby's father was seventeen; when La Shana Lewis became pregnant, she was fifteen and her baby's father was eighteen. The greatest gap was between fifteen-year-old Cassandra Witt and the baby's twenty-six-year-old father, making him the oldest father in this group. He was also married, much to Cassandra's chagrin—something she did not know until she was pregnant.

Twenty-nine teen fathers lived with their single mothers and siblings. Five were high school students. Two had taken college courses. Over half of the teen fathers worked at low-skilled jobs, such as truck driver's assistant, furniture mover, construction worker, and janitor during their relationships with the teen girls. Some of the teen mothers knew that a few teen fathers were involved in illegal activities, such as selling drugs or petty crimes. Regardless of the father's source of income, most of the teen mothers said they did not receive or expect any support—financial or otherwise—from these men.

Several older teen mothers declared they had been involved with the teen fathers for almost three years. Margaret Thompson spent five "wonderful" years with a man who abruptly ended the relationship when she told him she was pregnant. On average, though, most of the teen mothers had stories similar to that of Terry Parks: a year-long involvement that ended as soon as the pregnancy was confirmed.

Terry Parks

Alma Harris, Diane's middle-class, image-conscious mother, would say that Terry Parks's history fit those ghetto-mentality teen mothers she disliked so much. But Terry, a slightly built eighteen-year-old mother whose eyes twinkled when she smiled, did not quite fit that assessment. She shared a tiny, two-bedroom apartment in East Oakland with her two-year-old son Cecil and twenty-year-old Dana Little and Dana's five-year-old son. When Terry and Dana approached their social workers to suggest they could become roommates, the workers told them that welfare regulations prohibited two AFDC families from sharing lodgings. The two mothers disagreed with the regulation. Their lives would be much easier if they could share expenses and child care.

Terry and Dana found a quiet apartment building on a street of mostly single-family homes. They turned their apartment into a cozy home, despite its small size. They painted the dingy walls white, scrubbed the floors until they gleamed, hung red and white checked kitchen curtains, and taped their children's drawings to the refrigerator door. To keep their shared housing arrangement a secret from the social worker, they developed elaborate procedures to collect mail and receive phone calls at a friend's home. It was worth it, Terry said, as she took me on a tour of the apartment: "I feel very comfortable here."

Terry told Dana that we planned to have a private interview, but Dana, who was all smiles and apologies as she pulled tussling Damon and Cecil apart, ignored her request. After coaxing the children to play in a narrow space behind the sofa, Dana took a seat in the chair across from us. She became an unofficial, but welcome, presence in the interview, offering opinions on everything from men to abortion. The children interrupted us numerous times, but somehow we managed to talk about the mothers' families, problems with AFDC, and the babies' fathers.

Terry herself had been the baby of a teenage mother who had had to apply for AFDC because her mother could not give her financial assistance. Terry's mother remembered what it was like being a teenage mother. She told Terry she would not force her to move. Terry did move, however, because she needed more space and a chance to become an independent person. She gave her mother credit for being emotionally supportive, for giving her helpful information about her own pregnancy, and for letting her know how happy she was when Terry was born.

Terry described an ordinary childhood filled with friends and school activities. Although her family never had enough food or clothing, life was tolerable. She had been a skinny, short, plain little girl. Then, almost over night, there was a different person in the mirror. Gesturing widely as she talked, Terry described how she changed from an "ugly duckling" into a pretty teenager, a few inches taller with bigger "boobs."

Suddenly—at least it seemed that way to Terry—shortly before her thirteenth birthday the boys in the school yard began talking to her, walking her home, and telling her how cute she looked. Just after celebrating her fourteenth birthday, Terry had DeWayne's attention: "I was going to school, and he was coming up to the school all the time to pick up his friend. His friend was talking to my friend. So he picked her up and he picked me up. He dropped me off at my home and it was like, 'What's your name?' And I introduced myself. We went for rides and stuff and he finally said, 'I want to meet your parents.' He met my mother." His attention to the courtship ritual of meeting her mother set DeWayne apart from the other boys she knew. Soon they were eating lunch together, borrowing tape cassettes from each other, and sitting on park benches with their arms intertwined.

Terry did not feel pressured by DeWayne to have sex; she had sex because of her strong emotional feelings for DeWayne and her belief that he felt the same way: "I never felt loved this way before. Everyone else had always let me down, disappointed me: 'Oh I'm going to do this for you and that for you.' And they never come through. This was the first time I ever experienced being loved by a man."

She was in love and assumed he meant it when he said he was too. But the talk of love between Terry and DeWayne, spoken in the same language, had different meanings to the two adolescents. Terry's relationship with DeWayne only lasted nine months. One afternoon, as Terry was dressing to see a movie with DeWayne, her mother reminded her of her annual doctor's appointment. She was only a month late, she told herself—no need to worry. Later that afternoon, the doctor confirmed she was one month pregnant. This day, she remembered not her own feelings but her mother's anger: "She was so angry. I was crying, telling my momma, 'Momma, Momma, I'm going to have it.' And I started crying and I just grabbed her and hugged her. She didn't say nothin'. And then we got home and she was trying to convince me to have an abortion."

At first Terry wanted to have an abortion, but events pulled her in another direction. A week after she told DeWayne the news, he dropped by her house: "At first he really didn't say anything, just sat there, and then he asked what did I plan on doing and I said I planned on having it. He said he didn't think it was a good idea and that I was still young and I should have an abortion." Terry was surprised. She thought they were close.[1] After all, they had been seeing each other for almost a year. Why would he not support her in whatever decision she made about the pregnancy? After many sleepless nights, she decided to do what DeWayne and her mother wanted. Her mother made the arrangements. DeWayne and her mother agreed to share the two-hundred-dollar clinic fee. On the day of the appointment, she waited and waited for him. "He never brought the money by." Terry remembered her mother calling DeWayne's house, talking to his father, and becoming angry when she learned he didn't know about Terry's pregnancy. His father told her that DeWayne was not at home. He had gone off to visit his cousin in Atlanta, Georgia. Terry could not believe he would leave her. She called that day "bad luck day": "And I said, 'Forget it. I'm going to have my baby.' Then one day, two weeks later, he called me. He told me it ain't his and all that stuff. And he asked me what I was going to do. And I said, 'I'm going to have it.' He just got mad and hung up."

Terry's mother, Eleanor Parks, perhaps recalling her own early experiences, pleaded with her daughter to save her reputation by marrying DeWayne. Terry loved him, but she also had an image of marriage as a white wedding dress, a fancy wedding, and happiness ever after. She could not overcome this romantic notion just to salvage her reputation. Terry was so ashamed about being pregnant that she dropped out of school so her friends would not find out. Since most of her friends were her schoolmates, the soon-to-be mother effectively isolated herself from the other girls her age. She did not realize how badly she would feel about it later.

DeWayne did see Terry again. After the baby's birth he occasionally visited her home. One afternoon he told her that the baby looked like one of his friends. He told his mother the same story, Terry believed. Shortly after that visit he brought his mother to see the baby only to have his mother say, "Yeah, it looks like you," before walking out to leave him standing awkwardly in the living room.

Dana told a similar story. In two other cases she knew of, the paternal grandmothers confirmed the identity of the babies' fathers on the basis of facial resemblance. The grandmother's declaration of DeWayne's fatherhood helped Terry feel better about her situation, but it did not make DeWayne more involved with his son. He stopped by Terry's apartment only occasionally. He refused to give her any money, because, he said, she might spend it on herself. She said she became resigned to his attitude. Her words, almost a whisper, were slow and hesitant:

And now it's like we don't get along. The baby asks for his daddy, and what should I tell him? That he takes what happens out on me by not coming around, by not buying him anything? Just being real angry with me because when he called me once, he wanted to have sex and I said, 'No!' (loud voice). It hurts me and I hold it in. But it hurts because I haven't seen him but I can't keep my son from asking, "Mommy, when am I going to see my daddy?"

I did get angry at first. But nothin' I can do. Cecil's going to ask me about him and I'm going to tell him.

He Loved Me Until I Got Pregnant

Other teen mothers expressed similar feelings of hurt and betrayal when they talked about their babies' fathers. Lois Patterson sat across from me in a small, airless family room. Her husky voice rose as she spoke about the beginning and end of her relationship with the baby's father:

He asked me would I be his lady. And I said yeah. And we went to his house. I did it for the first time and got pregnant. I said, "I ain't takin' nothin' so we shouldn't do that." And he said, "I ain't gonna let nothin' happen." Then he liked me. We use to go to the movies.[2]

Now he can't stand me. Claims he can't. He didn't have nothin' to say to me. 'Cause he was mad because I was pregnant. He wanted me to have an abortion. I told him no. I wasn't havin' no abortion. I asked him, "When the baby gets here, what you goin' to do?" He said he was going to feed the baby Gravy Train dog food.

—*So the relationship stopped when you told him you were pregnant?*

Yeah. He said, "It ain't mine."

—*How did you feel when he said that?*

Oh, I was mad. But I said, "Hmm." I was hurt. But I said, "Well."

—*Did you cry?*

Nope. No! He said that I got pregnant by my sister's old man. Yeah, that's what he told me. I laughed. "Boy, you're funny." I said, "Are you going to tell your mother?" And he said, "I ain't going to tell her nothin' (voice in a whisper). I said, "That's cool."

But the tremor in her voice betrayed her: she did not really think it was cool. Lois, who will later say that she did not expect anything from her baby's father, was stunned by his treatment of her: "He didn't help me when I was pregnant. He didn't pay me no mind. And we use to go to the same school. I'd see him at the bus stop I'd walk down. I'd let him catch the bus first and I'd get the other bus . . ." Lois stopped in mid-sentence.

Other teen mothers were equally dismayed when the fathering role did not materialize. Seventeen-year-old Jackie Marley and eighteen-year-old Annie Blake had similar stories. Annie added, "He won't come around, and her birthday is the same day as his." Annie and I were sitting at a small kitchen table, squeezed in between the stove and the refrigerator. The sounds of the radio and children's voices drifted in from the living room, making it difficult to have a conversation. I wished she had a private bedroom. She was really not "getting along fine." She was having problems getting AFDC, and she was failing school because she could not study and take care of her baby at the same time. She could not stay with her mother because they argued all the time, so she slept at the homes of relatives and friends.

Shirley Foster Hartley finds that teenage fathers generally express negative attitudes and behavior toward the teenage mothers. Hartley concludes that the fathers' negativism may stem from their feelings of insecurity about fatherhood: "Flight into purely pseudoadulthood [through sex] can be dangerous to all concerned," when youthful identity problems are aggravated by parenthood. Hartley uses the term *pseudoadulthood* to reflect her belief that these adolescents may feel so threatened by the tremendous responsibility of being fathers at such a young age that they try to resolve these feelings by "devising derogatory stereotypes about the unwed mothers."[3] Carlo Salguero's study on adolescent fathers suggests that over half of Black adolescent fathers stop seeing the mothers of their babies three months after the babies' births.

Margaret Thompson, an attractive forty-year-old secretary, sat on a lumpy sofa in a crowded employees' lounge for two hours one sweltering summer afternoon to talk about her baby's father. She had conducted a two-year search to find him so that she could collect child support, and she had decided to give it up only recently. Now, happily married and the mother of another child, she shuddered at the memories of that relationship: "And, of course, when I told him I was pregnant, that was all over with. At the time he worked for General Motors. He made real good money. It must have been nine dollars an hour. And he was just interested in his life and his things that he couldn't really get into it. He denied everything. He just moved. I was hurt being alone and having a baby. So fuck him. And then I started wanting to have the baby."

"Why?" I asked.

As she stood up to return to her office, Margaret said, "Because it would be mine. It was the first time I would have something to love and that would love me back. He loved me until I got pregnant."

Margaret Thompson's answer reinforced Hartley's assertion that when the baby's father withdraws his emotional support, "The unwed mother may even expect the growing child to provide emotional support for her."[4]

Love and Commitment

"What did you expect from the baby's father?" I asked each of the thirty-two teen mothers. The following six responses are typical:

Terry Parks:	I told him, "I don't want nothin' from you—just take care of your responsibilities."
Susan Carter:	Well, I expect him to be there for my daughter. I expect him, if me and him don't work out, no matter how much I hate him, I'm never gonna stop him from seeing his daughter. I want him to pay child support. That's definite. He's going to pay child support.
Diane Harris:	I expected commitment of just being a father. Of being there saying, "I'm going to help you, I'll be there to take care of Jimmy when you want, when you need to do other things." I expected his support emotionally, financially, as much as he could. I expected him to love me because I was the woman who had his baby. But he loves everyone else who didn't.
Shana Leeds:	I expected him to be helpful: take care of the baby. All three of us go places and have fun. Live together as a family.
Lois Patterson:	Really nothin'.
De Vonya Smalls:	That maybe we would talk about it if I said I was going to keep it.

The mothers' words reveal two kinds of expectations: one regarding their own relationships, the other the babies' relationships with the teen fathers. Each mother expected something different from her relationship with the baby's father. De Vonya wanted a relationship based on mutual support. Most important to Diane, who was very clear about it, was that the baby's father needed to act like a father. Unlike De Vonya and Diane, Shana Leeds saw the three of them as a family. Lois Patterson said she wanted "nothin'," but this disclaimer would prove to be false.

Like motherhood, fatherhood consists of a set of norms that men as fathers are expected to follow. Although these men were biologically fathers, they failed to live up to the teen mothers' view of fatherhood. The teen mothers believed that fathers should love, guide, protect, and provide for their children. Based on those assumptions about fatherhood, most of the teen mothers (except Lois Patterson) thought the men would jump over any hurdle in their lives to care for their children. Or, if their relationship ended, the men would still adhere to the fatherhood mandate. For instance, Susan, perhaps predicting an end to her affair with Joney, talked about her need for him to be a good father regardless of the outcome of their relationship.

All Those Lies: Diane Harris

In her expectations of the baby's father, Diane Harris pushed for middle-class values wrapped up in the American Dream of family life—something she had watched her family strive to obtain. But Diane's current lifestyle contrasted greatly with that of her early childhood in the family's home in the Oakland hills.

Diane's apartment building in North Oakland looked like all the others I had visited in the past months. Diane greeted me at the door dressed in a bathrobe; she had forgotten about our morning appointment. Two hours earlier, at seven, she had gotten up, given Jimmy Jr. some crackers, and put him in front of the television so that she could go back to sleep. As I watched her, I thought about the popular view of teen mothers. How easy it would be for me to see this young mother, who stood at the door casually dressed in a bathrobe while her son watched cartoons in the living room, as the stereotypical

Black teenage mother. Yet nothing could be further from the truth. Diane, a firm believer in mainstream values, was an outspoken critic of what she referred to as the "ghetto mentality" of teenage welfare mothers.

Diane's apartment was certainly more splendid than the other teen mothers' homes. The rooms looked polished and slick, and every space was filled with contemporary furniture. In the two bedrooms long white window drapes fell gracefully to the floor and large framed posters lined the freshly painted walls. "Never mind" all the sharp furniture, she told me, when I complimented her on the apartment's appearance. Diane explained that the furnishings were some gifts from her mother, who was trying to make it up to her for treating her so badly during her pregnancy. They do not make up for the loneliness she feels: "I want somebody to love me and to want to take care of me emotionally and financially. I wish that, but it's not too bad. I do have a nice place to live."

At first she thought life with Jimmy Weber would be like life with her father. She believed "all those lies," she sighed. She said she was too young and too sheltered to know that he was not sincere when he said he loved her. Living with him, a man who offered little emotional support, was "nothing but a problem." The young mother folded her arms across her chest as she talked. "He stayed out all night. He gave out our telephone number to women who called the house all the time. One of his girl friends had the nerve to send me a get well card when I was sick." She laughed at the memory.

She began to realize that with Jimmy she would not have the warm, comfortable family home of her childhood, the kind of life in which vacations to the Bahamas were possible and where Christmases were spent skiing in Colorado. He would never be a good father nor a good husband. "Runaround types never are," she explained. Jimmy could not give her the kind of life she had before she met him:

He had a ghetto mentality. He's the kind of person who likes a casual living style. I want to get as far away as possible from this life, even if it means giving up my son. My fantasy is to give him to his father, to get married, to live somewhere else, like in another state. To marry a professional, someone who has values and ideals like I have. Have more children, be a corporate attorney, have a big beautiful house, and a car. Have money. Have four children, all with my husband. Raise them and send them to college. There's a real good sense of self-worth in that.

Although I felt that Diane's fantasy about her son was just talk, it weighed heavily enough on her mind to make her bring up the subject several times. She felt trapped in a bad relationship with a child who might ruin her chances of improving her class, of marrying a man who could give her back what she lost when she became pregnant. She would probably disagree with my assessment. She professed to being more sensitive than her mother, but her fantasy allowed her to relive her mother's notions about class status and image.

Fantasy aside, Diane was also worried that Jimmy would leave her for another woman. Diane felt Jimmy was her only marriage possibility because she had an illegitimate child. Several months after our interview she did marry Jimmy. In a way, a feminist perspective could argue, this relationship had really encompassed both her emotional needs and Jimmy's. She wanted and needed love. The gendered norms she was expected to follow required that she value the integrity of their relationship more than he. She placed emotional commitment to him higher on her list of moral values than she thought he did. He had to serve his emotional needs first, she believed, and that involved the desire to be sexually active as a way of defining his masculinity.

Two Different Worlds

Love and long-term commitment—words in Diane's dreams. Teenage mothers' dreams of love, family, and commitment to another teenager seem like pipe dreams in light of the changeable agendas of adolescents. Since the teen mothers' and fathers' backgrounds were so similar and their relationships lasted for at least a year, the teen mothers did not see the different meanings they made of relationships. Nor did they realize that they lived in a gender-segregated world. Romance novels, popular magazines, and soap operas confirm these teenagers' image of love. However, as I suggest, and the sociological literature supports, these young mothers associate sex with love, while the teen men think of sex only as part of the masculine quest.

Sometimes during my visits with the teen mothers I had a chance to browse their bookshelves. The most widely read materials were popular magazines such as *Essence* and *Ebony*. Several of the articles in *Essence* were about eligible men venting their feelings about women and fatherhood. These articles had provocative titles: "When My Economic Status Fell, My Relationships with Women Started to Suffer," "If I Become a Father, I'm Afraid I May Not Prove Strong and May Run Away."[5] The men quoted in the *Essence* articles said they left relationships because they earned too little. The women in this study saw it differently, and that difference in perceptions of their shared worlds speak volumes about their gender relations.

To understand why women see love and commitment this way, Carol Gilligan suggests that we need to understand that "women's sense of integrity appears to be entwined with an ethic of care, so that to see themselves as women is to see themselves in a relationship of connection."[6] Two teen mothers' fantasies contained elements of Gilligan's theory of caring:

Diane: I want to live in a big house with Jimmy Jr., and I want to have nice things in life. And I wanna have somebody, more than anything. I don't want to live by myself. I want somebody that's going to be a good father to [my baby].

Terry: My fantasy is that after I get married, go off somewhere, far off to myself, just me and my little family.

Diane's and Terry's fantasies of the good life included a "big house" and a "little family." Commitment, family, and a father for their children were high on that list.

The Masculine Mandate

Several problems with Diane's and Terry's fantasies of the good life, which included fathers for their babies, made them unachievable. For years sociologists have convincingly argued that the tremendous problems Black men confront in a racist labor market make it difficult, and sometimes impossible, for them to be good husbands and fathers. Black men are forced into low-paying jobs or onto unemployment lines, or unemployment forces them into a life of crime, drugs, homicide, or suicide. As William J. Wilson and others note, these Black men have little opportunity to fulfill men's primary family obligations. These family obligations are related to what Jessie Bernard calls the "good provider" responsibility. Bernard asserts, "The good provider is a family man. He sets a good table, provides a decent home, pays the mortgage, buys the shoes, and keeps his children warmly clothed."[7]

However, the American economic structure favors White men, especially those of the middle class. Therefore, Jessie Bernard's model of the good provider works for them and a few Black men, like Evie Jenkins's and Diane Harris's middle-class fathers, while most Black men are isolated from the mainstream labor market.[8] This problem is felt acutely by Black men, since men's ability to earn a living is linked to their masculinity. According to this masculine mandate, real men provide quite well for their wives and children. Consequently, as Robert Staples explains it, Black men "have never been given the opportunities of manhood—life-sustaining employment and the ability to support a family." Staples's study examines the connection between Black men's employment and the family and concludes, "The opportunities to perform at this critical task are less available for Black men than for many non-Black men; the lack of steady jobs is particularly acute for young Black men."[9]

Given their socioeconomic history, then, I was not surprised to hear that some teen fathers (and the teen mothers' own fathers) were in jail, had died young, or, though not in jail, were involved in crime and drugs. Troy Duster describes these men as being at the "base of the American economy and policy." But sociologist Daniel Thompson adds an emotional component to this discussion of Black men as providers. He observes that while their lack of economic opportunity may derive from situations "external to them," they feel seriously affected by their failure to provide for their families. Other studies find that these men often become so ashamed of their failure that they leave their families and take to the streets, where they surround themselves with other unemployed men.[10]

These explanations of Black men's absence from their families, while important and insightful, do not go far enough. As I noted earlier, the teen mothers suggested that some of the teen fathers worked and could have provided some financial or emotional support.

Some feminists stress the idea that most boys, regardless of race, ethnicity, or class, devalue girls. Their research shows that quite often boys are born into a world that values them more than it values girls.

(Terry Parks and her roommate discuss this very important point in Chapter 6.) Very early in boys' lives, they learn to see girls as objects and to emphasize sex. These feminist authors point to research on gender that finds children as young as two years old aware of their gender and adhering to gender stereotypes.[11]

Elizah Anderson makes a similar point. He argues persuasively that the sexual conquest of women becomes more important to men than commitment. Anderson quotes a seventeen-year-old teenage father who told him that boys go as far as "pulling a game" on the young love-starved girls to win them over: "Yeah, they'll take you out. Walk you down to Center City, movies, window shop [laughs]. They point in the window. 'Yeah, I'm gonna get this. Wouldn't you like this? Look at the nice livin' room set.' Then they want to take you to his house, go to his room: 'Let's watch some TV.' Next thing you know is your clothes is off and you in the bed havin' sex, you know."[12] Anderson calls this teenager a "gamesman." He notes, "The young men variously describe their successful campaigns and conquests as 'getting over.'" In order to "get over," the young men devise and develop a "game," whose success is gauged by its acceptance by both his peers and by young women. The game consists of a full presentation of a sham self, including dress, grooming, and conversation, or "rap." The men are exceedingly good at this "game" of conquest, Anderson believes. But they do not care about the women. They really desire sex without commitment, and when they impregnate a girl, they will produce babies without taking on the responsibility for them.

Partners: The Male Culture of Protection

De Vonya Smalls patted her baby to sleep as she talked about Matthew, the baby's father. Although they had been together for a year when she became pregnant, he told her to have an abortion. When she refused, he stopped speaking to her. She found it especially difficult to handle his snubs when her friends were with her in the school yard or in the school cafeteria and he walked by as if she did not exist. Despite his treatment of her, and with her usual display of wisdom, De Vonya offered reasons for Matthew's behavior: "He was young and he was scared."

De Vonya's baby's father would fit Diane Harris's "ghetto mentality" profile of lower-class Black men. But DeVonya's description of Matthew's reaction revealed the influence of the male peer group, similar to the reactions of the men in Anderson's study.[13] De Vonya thought that Matthew's friends had turned against her, forming a "culture of protection" around him, which allowed him to evade his responsibility to her and their baby: "He wouldn't have nothing to do with me after he find out I was pregnant. I think it's his so-called friends, his partners, what they be tellin' him: 'Well, man, that's not your baby, you shouldn't take care of that baby.' And all of that." De Vonya called Matthew's friends "partners" to indicate that each person in the peer group had an investment in the others' lives.

According to Anderson, the boys are careful not to become seriously involved with the girls. If they do become involved, they could be considered "pussywhipped" by their friends.[14] This notion is based on the assumption that "real men" do not become emotionally involved—an old sexist and homophobic fear that equates emotion with femininity. Sexism and homophobia are thus useful male peer strategies in the "game." The Black male gamesmanship discussed by Anderson seems no different from that of White men, who see women in the same way. Anderson also assumes that "gamesmen" end their "gamesmanship" at an appropriate time in their lives. The major problem, however, with Anderson's analysis of these men who prove their masculinity through sexual conquest is that it does not question how that perception of masculinity developed in the first place and who ultimately pays for their sexual relations.

If gender learning begins at an early age and has such a tremendous impact on boys and girls, it may be extremely difficult, although not impossible, for men to unlearn their "gamesmen" strategy at the appropriate time. Men take their cues about masculinity from the dominant view that men are more valued than women. In fact, an understanding of the dynamics of Black masculine identity can unravel the dominant masculine ideology itself. As Noel Cazanave puts it, "The hopes, aspirations, attitudes, and behaviors of men are formed in this process of masculine attainment, and its vicissitudes are a major motivating force behind much of the day-to-day interactions and lifestyles of American males."[15]

In Chapter 1 I noted that the teenage fathers were difficult to interview; nonetheless, the gendered world of these young men and women was visible to me in several ways. I could occasionally witness several babies' fathers interacting with the teen mothers. The one that stood out the most revealed how some of these men tried to impose their authority even in fatherless homes. Eighteen-year-old Jermain Trainer refused to participate in this study. Although he was always too busy to visit De Lesha Simons and their baby, he did call her occasionally. When she told him that she wanted to be interviewed for this study, even without his participation, he told her, "No way." The determined seventeen-year-old mother consented to be interviewed anyway. "I wanted a chance to tell my story."

On the day of the interview, Jermain barged into the apartment, brushing past De Lesha's mother, who asked him to leave. Ignoring her, he pushed open the door to De Lesha's bedroom, where we sat. He struck a menacing pose in the doorway and demanded that she help him search for a sweater he had left behind. When I offered to help her find the sweater, he mumbled, "We can do it later," and quickly walked out. De Lesha Simons concluded, "He wanted to check you out." He was satisfied that I did not pose a threat to him or to her. I did not tell her I suspected that he was involved with drugs and his real motive may have been to see whether I was an investigator.

Jermain could walk freely into De Lesha Simons's house, Anderson would argue, because he perceived the women in that household to have little authority. To quote Anderson, "The male authority figures as agents of social control cannot be overestimated."[16] As Anderson sees it, the presence of the father in the home of a teenage girl was and is an important factor in determining whether the boy respects the girl and her family. It seems to me that the father's gender has less to do with his situation than the perception of the men's power. As Anderson admits, women can also gain that kind of authority. Two decades ago the old neighborhood women (as they were commonly referred to) were able to assert their authority over the girls and the boys they knew.

The teen mothers did not see their relationships as games. They talked about the practical and emotional price they paid for being involved with these men. A study on the short- and long-term impact of teenage pregnancy on parents' education, occupation, and marital and childbearing lives finds that it is the teenage mothers, not the teenage fathers, who lose out.[17] As Anderson observes, the teen mothers are vulnerable to "brief liaisons" with men who have a choice of sexual partners and are not interested in marriage or parental commitment.[18] Indeed, one effect of the "game" on the teen mothers was the limits it placed on the emotional support they so desperately needed.

Child Support Problems

Both De Vonya and Terry were so hurt, angry, and humiliated by the babies' fathers that they could not bring themselves to ask for financial support.[19] In fact, Terry knew where her baby's father lived and De Vonya saw her baby's father every day at school. But De Vonya was so offended by Matthew's treatment of her that she refused to tell anyone, not even her mother, about him. Terry told her mother about DeWayne, but she wanted nothing else to do with him.

There is an added dimension to the issue of child support. Lois Patterson's baby's father refused to pay child care support, although he had two jobs: "He's a baker, and he's a meat cutter." When his son was first born, he refused to see Lois, but he then began to visit the teen mother's house weekly to see the baby. When he adamantly refused to contribute any money for child care, Lois began to think that his visiting was a scheme to pretend to be involved with the baby to avoid paying child support. In discussing her baby's father, she fell back on the old cultural norm about fathers: "They should give money as well as love their kids." If they did not provide money, she implied, they should not be allowed to offer love instead. Two years after the baby's birth the baby's father was ordered by the court to pay three hundred dollars a month in back child support payments. Furious, he reduced his visits with his son. Lois said: "That's why he's mad. And so he stopped comin'. He came by on his birthday and brought him a skateboard. I told him not to buy him one and he went out and bought him one anyway. But he don't come by like he use to do—take him out for dinner and get his hair cut or take him to a movie. He hates this."

Other teen fathers may have hated paying child support. Two other teen mothers had to obtain child support through the court. Carita

Hughes shook her head in bewilderment at the "embarrassing court scene" that took place when her baby's father told the judge he did not father her child; she had to have the baby's blood tested to win child support. "It was all for nothing," Carita said. The day following the court decision, she learned that the father quit his job and disappeared.

Terry Parks and Dana Little listened intensely as I told them about such experiences. Dana could hardly wait to tell us her "diaper story":

After the baby was born, the baby's father came by once. And once I went to him. I happen to live three blocks away from him, and asked, "Hey, this is my last Pamper, and I don't want to have to ask you for anything, but I have to ask you for money for diapers." And he was really funny about it (her voice was nervous). He ran in the house. I waited outside for two hours. I guess he thought I would leave, you know. He gave it, but he made me keep asking, made me sweat for it.

This teen father had a job. Maybe he did not make "big bucks," but Dana wanted to know why he made her "sweat" (she repeated the word several times) for the diaper money.

Denise Collins suggested another reason some men refuse to pay child support. When asked why her baby's father did not visit or support her son, she said softly, "He has so many children that my son is just one more."

Strategies of Resistance

Earlier in this chapter I said that the teen mothers expected and hoped that the babies' fathers' commitment to them would resolve any tension between these men's interests and the mothers' needs. De Vonya and all the teens believed the teen fathers' commitment to them as mothers of their children would evolve naturally from the intimacy and history they shared. Instead, according to the teen mothers' perceptions, the teen fathers brought with them an unintegrated vision and culture of maleness in which proving their masculinity consumed their lives and women and men are not seen as functioning together. All of these factors can lead to relationships in which men and women (in this case, teen mothers and teen fathers) do not understand each other, do not communicate with each other, and are isolated from each other. This kind of gender-segregated lifestyle was apparent in the teen mothers' description of their poor relationships with the babies' fathers.

The women had a few strategies to maintain the link between them and the babies' fathers, despite the babies' fathers' treatment of them and the young mothers' refusal to ask the teen fathers for child support. Some of their strategies were creative and worked; others only reproduced the very gender inequality they discussed. There were strategies to force the men to acknowledge their fatherhood in order to undermine the babies' fathers attempts to completely forsake them. One was to have the paternal grandmothers recognize their sons' children. Another was to inform the fathers of the teen men about the pregnancies and the teen fathers' unsupportiveness. Another strategy to maintain the link between themselves and the teen fathers was to parade the babies around the teen fathers' friends when the fathers were not around, exclaiming, "Doesn't the baby look just like him?" By displaying the babies and pointing out the similarities of features, the teen mothers, in effect, winked at the fathers' denial, as if to say, "Come on now, we all know the truth." Indirectly, these teen mothers' strategies also told the teen fathers' friends that they were not defeated.

There were even more strategies: Dana's waiting outside her baby's father's apartment until he relented and gave her some diaper money; Lois's demanding that the baby's father pay money for child care. While one could argue that these strategies accomplished very little, the teen mothers did feel their strategies demonstrated to the teen fathers that they were much more than passive "good girls."

Other strategies did not work. By refusing to identify the father of her child, De Vonya protected herself from having to deal with him anymore. Both De Vonya and Terry allowed the babies' fathers to claim they were not the fathers, thereby supporting the fathers' goal of not providing them with child support. If legally forced to pay child support, as Lois's baby's father was, they stopped seeing their children. Only a few people—the teen mothers themselves and the mothers of some of the teen fathers—seemed offended by the way the men walked away so easily. No one mentioned to the teen fathers that given the girls' ages, especially that of fifteen-year-old Cassandra Witt (whose baby's father was twenty-six), they had committed a criminal act—statutory rape. Neither the teen mothers nor their mothers (nor the counselors at the Alternative Center) ever thought in those terms. What is at the root of such denial?

What about Terry Parks's own father? What did she mean when, in summing up her feelings about her baby's father, she told me the following: "I don't feel so bad. I mean growing up without a father is not the hardest thing in the world. I did it." What does this absence of both kinds of fathers in the lives of these young women explain? Are there connections to be made between their absence and the teen mothers' acceptance, like Terry's, of the absence of the teenage fathers?

Chapter Six

The Teens' Fathers

It's not much to say about my father.
Sixteen-year-old Georgia Minns

"What about your father?" I finally asked Terry Parks one afternoon. During the hour she had talked quite freely about her mother and DeWayne but had not even mentioned her father: "He was in jail a lot. He died last year. I saw him every blue moon." Like Terry, most of the teen mothers said they knew almost nothing about their fathers' ages or residences or where they worked. Twenty-two of the teen mothers said, "I don't know," to questions about their fathers' backgrounds. Sixteen-year-old Carmilla Hopkins lowered her voice to a whisper when she said, "I don't know my father. I've never even seen a picture of him." Her tone of voice implied that she was not angry at him but that she had simply accepted this situation, although perhaps with a sense of shame or disappointment.

Even Susan Carter, who spent nearly fourteen years with her father, admitted with some embarrassment: "I don't know if he has a job or anything. I don't know how old my father is, I don't. I've never asked any questions of him." Interestingly, she did not ask her mother or any other relatives about her father, either. Nor did her mother volunteer any information about her daughter's father.

The few teen mothers who did talk about these men drew sketches of threadbare, painful relationships. The teen mothers described four types of fathers. Most were described as "walk away" fathers, who had no contact with their daughters. "Every blue moon" fathers moved in and out of their daughters' lives willy-nilly. "Uninvolved" fathers lived at home but had little presence in their daughters' lives. Only five teen mothers described the fourth type of father, who was actively or "somewhat" engaged in their lives. The first three categories of fathers are striking not only in and of themselves but also because they describe the teen fathers as well. For example, Terry Parks said her father "walked away"; so did her baby's father. Shana Leeds referred to both her father and her baby's father as "every blue moon" types. Evie Jenkins's father was present but uninvolved. She said the same about her baby's father. Diane Harris's father, who had died several years before, was one of the few who had served as a loving, supportive father; Diane's son's father was somewhat involved in his life. Class differences between the teen mothers seemed to play a role in their perceptions of their fathers. For example, the mothers who were poor tended to describe their fathers as being less supportive than the middle-class mothers.

More important issues were at play here than just categorizing these men as supportive or unsupportive. This chapter explores the meaning the teen mothers made of these pivotal relationships. The teenagers' statements questioning the importance of fathers in their lives also raised questions germane to the changing shape of Black families. As I noted in Chapter 1, the history of Black families in America is one of changing structures. The post–World War II nuclear family became the extended family of the 1970s. By the 1980s almost half of all Black families were headed by low-income women. This rise in women-headed households led many people to say that the Black family structure was deteriorating.

The two-parent household, so common as the ideal family model, is a cultural form based mainly on a Eurocentric patriarchal model of the family. The teen mothers unknowingly drew on this model when they discussed their family life, and by doing so they reinforced the gender, race, and class divides. Perhaps they did so because in the popular view, the female family form was deviant and necessary only when the patriarchal model was unobtainable; certainly some scholars on the Black community think so. The teen mothers expressed similar views. For example, Terry and Dana, who did not have positive alternative models of the family, grabbed onto the male-centered one and used it to gauge themselves, their fathers, and their mothers. These teen mothers' discussions of their fathers do pose a number of important questions that should be addressed in further studies on fathers.

Walk-Away Fathers

Two years before Cecil was born, Terry Parks became curious about her father's whereabouts. She asked everyone she knew about him, including her mother, who had never discussed this man who "dumped" her the same year Terry was born. Then one day she met him:

—Did he come by to see you?

No. He happened to see me and my mother on the street walking somewhere.

She was dismayed that they may have passed each other often on the street all those years without her knowing it. Almost immediately she began to gather information about him. One day she decided to meet him again. She looked up his address in the telephone book:

So when I found out, I went over there and I met him and my aunt, his side of the family. And then we started keeping in touch. He went to jail a short time later. I started writing him while he was in jail.

—How did he respond to your writing him and keeping in touch with his family?

Surprised. He was happy that I was finally able to meet my grandmother.

—Did he explain why he hadn't kept in touch with you?

Just, "I'm glad you're writing now." He didn't talk about the past. I didn't even want to talk about the past.

—Why didn't you?

What's done is done. I mean, it's nothin' I can do. Just, "Let's try to get to know each other now."

Was she afraid that he would leave again? Whatever the reason, Terry decided not to push him with questions about his absence. Did she expect anything of her father? "No," she said. "I wouldn't know what to expect from a father." Yet when I asked her and the other teen mothers about the kinds of fathers daughters should have, in interview after interview they spelled out very clearly the kind of father they would want. Without noticing the contradiction of her earlier statement, Terry said it best: "I know they're suppose to treat them right. Do for them, take them out, and treat them right, show them little things like how to use the bathroom or sports. My grandfather died when I was real young. So I never really had a real father. And my uncle that stayed with us once. My mother did all the work. So I've never really had a man around me. I don't need one. I get all my support from other people."

Did Terry's bathroom and sports references signal a nongendered view of what fathers should do for their daughters? Or was she perhaps thinking about the father of her son and what she wants him to do? The most significant point she made about fathers, which the others echoed, was the comment, "I don't need one."

I heard this remark again from another group of teen mothers at the Alternative Center's peer group meeting, where they met once a week to talk about personal issues. These teen mothers also did not think fathers were so important. After all, eighteen-year-old Annie Blake said, she had managed to live without one all these years. "What's the big deal?" she asked the group.

De Vonya Smalls also said, in a sad voice, that fathers were unimportant and unnecessary. After all, her baby's father wanted nothing to do with her or his baby, and she did not remember when her own father ever lived with her family. These feelings seemed to contradict her description of the tremendous effort she put into taking her baby on the BART train to Richmond in order to visit her father every Friday afternoon. Despite this effort, she complained, he did not return her visits: "Sometimes it gets on my nerves. 'Cause he's not doing the responsibility the way a father should, as old as he is. I try hard to make him more like a father, take me places, do things together." Once, hoping he would react, she stopped visiting him. He did not call to see if something was wrong. "He just don't care," she said in a flat voice. A month later she began to visit him again because, she said, he liked his granddaughter. She seemed to think she could make him "more like a father," by making him a grandfather.

Perhaps these "what's the big deal" comments and the teen mothers' limited knowledge about their fathers cover feelings of abandonment? If so, perhaps the strategy of not caring helped them deal with absent fathers. They seemed to say, "If Daddy is not around, it is because he doesn't care to be. So I will make him less important to me."

Every-Blue-Moon Father: Shana Leeds

Shana Leeds tried to make her father less important. She used the phrase "every blue moon" to situate first her baby's father and then her own father in her life. This phrase was part of the culture's language—all the teen mothers understood it. Shana, a mother at sixteen, lived in a low-income area of Richmond. She was in the ninth grade at an alternative school she attended for three hours a day. She was an emancipated minor; that is, she lived away from her family and was not supported by her parents. Each month she received $498 in AFDC benefits for her five-month-old daughter, Roselle. Food stamps were not included with her benefits. When I met Shana, she was living with a family friend. However, she insisted that we conduct the interviews at her mother's apartment because, as she put it, "The lady I live with don't like people coming to her house."

When I arrived at her mother's house, Shana led me into the living room of a neatly furnished two-bedroom flat filled with green plants and oversize furniture. Shana was wearing the popular teenage outfit: tight jeans, a long baggy print blouse, and black leather boots that stopped at her ankles. Her hair was cut in a short Afro that accented the slenderness of the shy and cautious teenager's face.

Shana's parents had separated when she was five years old. Shana shrugged her shoulders as she recalled her father's visits after her father and mother separated. Her mother kept the old frame house in East Oakland, and her father went to live in a small town outside Sacramento, where he remarried and had another daughter. Although he visited the Oakland area once or twice a year, he rarely saw Shana. Often he called with an excuse and a promise to see her the next time he was in the city.

She did not know much about him or what he did for a living. Every time she asked him about his job, he told her, "It's none of your business." Shana believed that he was afraid her mother would find out where he worked and try to collect child support from him. All Shana did know was, "I see him every blue moon. He doesn't live with us.

He just comes to visit every year, every two years. He has a job with the government. He won't come here. Not even now to see his grandson or me." Her mother, a nurse, supported Shana and her nine-year-old brother Michael until Shana moved out when her baby was born because the tension in the house became unbearable. She was constantly arguing with her mother over her refusal to marry Donnie, the baby's father: "I'm not going to marry someone who sees me only once in a while." He told her the baby was not his and stopped visiting her for several months: "One day he just popped up again. I saw him the last time a few days ago. I guess you could say he comes around every blue moon. You could say the same about my father."

Alicia Cummins used the same term as she recalled a father who waltzed in and out of her life: "I used to see my father once a summer. The last time was when he came to see me when the baby was born. She was two weeks old. He came again on Valentine's Day. But other than that, every blue moon." She seemed sad and regretful. Her voice trailed off as she looked down at her hands. In writing about father-daughter relationships, Linda Leonard states that a father's absence, "for whatever reason, due to death, war, divorce, or illness," is a condition of our culture and therefore shapes the structure of our lives. A real father, Leonard advises us, helps to shape his daughter's uniqueness and individuality, "but fathers can also hurt their daughters."[1] A father who leaves home by choice—the man who "loves 'em and leaves 'em"—may have a very negative emotional impact on his daughter. Further, as Lucy Rose Fischer observes, "It is the father's hierarchical position that makes his support particularly valuable."[2]

The teen mothers understood that these fatherly visits meant little. Sometimes the visits only increased the tension at home, adding to the teen mothers' beliefs that their fathers did not care much about them.

Shana's father did make the trip down to see her when he learned about her pregnancy. He "came over here trippin' and stuff," she said. "He got involved when my mother called him and told him I was pregnant. He came over here and met the baby's father. And he talked with him. Asked us, Is that what we wanted to do? and, What were we going to do when it gets here? How are we going to feed it? He kissed me and left. I don't know why he didn't give me no more support."

He did not ask her any questions about her life. "Just a peck on the cheek, and he was gone," she said. She didn't miss his insincerity: "It was all an act. He wants to demonstrate his manhood in front of another male." Shana perceived that her father's occasional visits were, in Goffman's terms, "a cover up," a "front" for his need to challenge the male authority of the baby's father, rather than interest in her well-being.[3] He merely passed as a father, without having emotional feelings for his daughter. She contrasted his coolness with her with her mother's anger: "She wanted to kill me."

Present But Uninvolved Fathers

Not all fathers left. Evie Jenkins's father had been home when she was a teenager, but she did not mention him in the interview. At first I had the impression that she grew up in a single-parent home. She had plenty of stories about her complex and troubling relationship with her mother, but nothing about her father. I learned about her father one afternoon when Debra May, Evie's daughter, joined one of our discussions. Debra May, tall and stout like her mother, had just celebrated her fifteenth birthday. Evie was concerned about her school problems. She was "earning a C when she could earn a B," Evie declared. She wanted me to give her daughter a motivational speech about the benefits of doing well in school. But Debra May was reluctant to talk about school because, she claimed, she hated her teachers.

Our discussion turned to the family. Debra May was more generous than her mother in sharing information about her grandfather, a man she loved a great deal. She thought her "grandmother's big mouth on everything" was the reason her grandfather did not say much about family matters. "He was basically a quiet, shy man," she said. "My grandmother's domineering ways didn't help."

Debra May's description of an overly controlling, strong and tough grandmother and a passive grandfather certainly matched the stereotypical picture of the bullying matriarch. Indeed, Evie's mother's strong presence was felt in our interview, while the man who had also lived with them had no presence at all. Still, the demanding grandmother description seemed too pat, fitting too easily the stereotype of "masculine" women. That image traces the faults of such a relationship to the woman's behavior or personality (a misogynist theory). It may also be that Evie's father's passivity forced Evie's mother to get "her big mouth on everything."[4]

Another way to view Evie's failure to provide information on her father is to consider it a deliberate strategy to counter her father's lack of involvement in her life. Other teen mothers also were silent about their fathers. Shana Leeds and De Vonya Smalls asked few questions about their fathers. Their attempts to replace such questions with assertions that fathers were not necessary or "no big deal" could be viewed also as a code of silence helping them handle the loss of their fathers.

Supportive Fathers

Only two teen mothers spoke fondly of their fathers. La Shana Lewis put it this way: "He's there when you need him. He doesn't talk that much. He listens a lot." "He's not like my mother," she said in a derogatory tone about her mother, whom she described as being "unsupportive." Such dichotomous thinking was very common among the teen mothers. Often they perceived their mothers as not being good mothers and their fathers as being very good, no matter how little they did or how often they were absent.

Diane Harris's father was very much involved in her life until he died a few years before. He was fully present in her memories as she recalled growing up in a comfortable, middle-class family where her father, whom she described as a "technical mechanic," devoted all his spare time to Diane. She spoke enthusiastically about him, emphasizing his good qualities. He was very special to her—a kind of Santa Claus figure. He loved her and was fun to be with, she said. He gave her a "more humane" set of values than her mother. He also gave her the sense that life was incomplete without a father: "Imagine your perspective of life if you don't have a father. All I saw was my father and it was very stable for me. I was raised by both my parents. I think most people know how life should be." She said, "His heart would break if he could see me now." According to Diane, her father spent his childhood in poverty, watching his mother struggling to clean offices at night and helping him with his homework during the day. He often told Diane that he still could empathize with people who were living in poverty. When he became a father, he vowed he would provide a stable family life for his children. She described her mother as a woman consumed with image and middle-class status and having little concern for people who were less fortunate.

The Halo Effect

In a society in which female-headed households are suspect, it is difficult for women to "give meaning" to their families in the way that fathers do, as Diane so nicely put it in referring to her father. The danger is, though, that men in short supply may be viewed as a high-demand commodity. If fathers are in high demand, one strategy might be to keep the memory of an absent father alive, as Diane did. Another strategy might be to replace the emotional impact of losing a father with compassion, as Terry did earlier. Terry did not become angry at her father for disappearing from her life or for living nearby and not contacting her. Instead, she transformed her anger at her father into understanding so that she could forgive him. Diane and Susan used other strategies to handle their feelings about their fathers. They describe their fathers as if a halo of male power surrounded them, thereby transforming them into models of perfection. Diane's father gave her a set of moral values she would treasure the rest of her life. Susan thought of her father as a powerful savior who could have prevented her from becoming pregnant. These teenagers used these strategies to restructure their emotional feelings so they could overlook their fathers' lack of involvement and then to create all-powerful fathers. Other examples of this replacement of emotional anger strategy came to mind when I asked Terry, "What did you think about all of this?" "It's best to forget about the past, to start over again. It don't bother me at all," she said, lowering her voice at the end. She mumbled under her breath, "It was time to chill out"—another cultural phrase I suspected had great significance to Terry. As part of that strategy of replacement of emotion, "chilling out" carried with it the connotation of handling strong emotions, of flattening them out, reshaping them, and then redirecting them onto the mother, keeping an unemotional stance toward the father in an effort to hold these emotions in check and below the surface. "It don't bother me at all," Terry sighed. This management of emotions required a great deal of effort to sustain.

As I said earlier, these teen mothers thought in dichotomous terms: "strong" or "good" fathers and "weak" or "bad" mothers. These daughters were so determined to have fathers that they obtained them at the expense of relationships with their mothers. Susan Carter was angrier at her mother for being unsupportive than at her father, who refused to see her. Only Terry Parks thought that her mother was supportive of her, yet in the section that follows, she will undermine that support. Shana Leeds muttered that she did not need a father, rerouting feelings of anger at and frustration with her father onto her mother, making this woman the center of her world, the culprit responsible for all her problems, perhaps because she was there and available.[5]

Diane Harris praised her father's values and degraded her mother's, and she angrily described her mother's perceived failures. Other teen mothers did the same. De Vonya Smalls, for instance, informed me that no matter how many problems her mother had, she was supposed to "be there" for her. De Vonya took a long bus trip every week to visit her noncommunicative father. Terry Parks was willing to forgive her long absent father for not visiting her. From her perspective, she had a good reason not to direct her anger at her father: the relationship was so tenuous. For all these teen mothers, it was almost as if they had to accept any kind of involvement from fathers, although they also admitted their fathers' failings: "Oh, he's just no good," or, "I didn't expect him to be there for me. He never is."

Constructing Daddy

When I compared Diane Harris's statements about her father with those of others who had different perceptions of their fathers, I realized that the teen mothers did indeed "know how life should be," as Diane suggested. From what they said about not needing fathers, it is clear that they did have a model of fathers in their minds. As we have just seen, they knew what fathers should be like and what they should do. How did they know, when so many of them had lived almost all their young lives without a father in their households and, judging from the numbers of Black families in similar situations, so had many of their friends? Like most other young American women, they said they took their model of the ideal father from the mainstream image of fathers.

Family life in America has been socially constructed around family holidays, family vacations, and family entertainment, and it is meant to include father, mother, and children. On Saturdays and Sundays, in many White and middle-class communities, such as where Diane Harris grew up, the playgrounds and parks are filled with fathers pushing swings or helping their children climb the jungle gym. While Father's Day is not revered in quite the same way as Mother's Day, most families do honor the responsible, hardworking, loving Dad who protects the family—especially "Daddy's little girls."

This image of a loving and hardworking father is reinforced by the media. During our discussion about the kind of father she wanted, Terry Parks told me about her fantasy dad. Most surprising, when I asked her where her ideas came from, she described the White father of *The Brady Bunch*, a television series popular in the 1970s: "To me, the Brady Bunch stands out. I remember watching them and thinking, 'What a nice family.' There was a man who was supportive and they all lived kinda nicely and nobody worried about money. The wife and husband always could be nice to their kids." Dana, Terry's roommate, interrupted Terry: "Me too." She also remembered watching the Brady Bunch and thinking, "Boy, what a swell life."[6]

That Terry accepted the media's image as reality is not surprising. According to James L. Caughey, in a society in which the media are an important entertainment source for so many, people may draw into their social network fictional characters they see every day. This fusion between the make-believe worlds of television and the real world occurs because, Caughey writes, "Individuals construct elaborate and enduring, albeit imagined relations with stars or with the characters they portray and turn to them for guidance and support." Caughey concludes, "Thus the attachments to unmet media figures [are] analogous to and in many ways directly parallel to actual social relationships with real 'fathers,' 'sisters,' 'friends' and 'lovers.'" These imaginary relations may have a decided impact on a person's self-esteem and may provide that person with an important source of advice and support. For example, someone who admires Mary Tyler Moore may deal with his or her own problems by wondering what Mary would do.[7]

In effect, television characters provided these teen mothers images of how people function in particular roles. The Brady Bunch father, a wise, gentle, and generous man, gave his family a large comfortable home and a funny maid who truly did seem like one of the family. Most of all, Mr. Brady loved his family. The Brady mother, neatly dressed, was always smiling and uncomplaining. They all lived nicely and did not have too many worries. The ones they did have were easily resolved, most often by Mr. Brady. Dana smiled, "And I said, 'Hey, I'm going to have that.'"[8]

The Brady Bunch family image not only told Terry and Dana what men were supposed to do as fathers but also showed them that the Bradys' lives were much more comfortable and stable than their own. The family life that the two teen mothers had managed to create, which could be disturbed at any moment if their social worker found them out, took place in quarters so cramped that their children's play area was confined to a foot of space between the sofa and the living room wall. Each month they worried about covering their living expenses, and they were never sure whether their babies' fathers would visit.

Several questions arose from Terry's and Dana's comments that pushed this analysis further. For example, why did these mothers use a father figure from old television reruns? Was there a thread running through these discussions of the Brady Bunch as a model of family life that linked Terry's search for her father with the idea that fathers were not needed? I began to compare Terry Parks's search for her father to that of adopted children who delve into the past to learn about their natural parents. All of them had the same reason to search for their parents: they wanted to round out their identities. Part of Terry's search for her father seemed to deal with unifying her total identity. Perhaps getting straight about her identity helped her gain control over some aspect of her life. Who she was and where she belonged in the world were crucial questions that gave her life historical and sociological significance.

Children ask questions about their identity all the time. "Where do you go to school?" "My mommy's and daddy's names are Hazel and George. What are your parents' names?" Other questions come up when boys and girls check their physical development against those of same-sex friends. "Am I as tall as you?" Children's questions about ethnicity and skin color are also ways to check identity. "Gabe's skin

color is different from mine. Why?" my son asked me when he confronted a playmate whose skin color was different from his.

All these questions are ways we as children learn to identify ourselves and our place in the world. If our search is successful, we develop a measure of security about ourselves. "See me," Terry could
say, having found some answers to sociological questions about herself. On the other hand, for teenagers like Terry, identification may be
complicated by issues of trust and security. For girls who grew up in
families with the father absent, the issues of identity are often not
predominantly issues of redefining and renegotiating family relationships but rather a search for a sense of where these girls are headed in
the future and the place they will take in society.[9]

If these teenagers were searching for their past and seeking information to help them gauge their future, we must ask another question. Why did these teenagers select a White television family like the
Bradys, and not the Huxtables, a Black middle-class television family,
as we might expect? Only three teen mothers said they identified with
the Huxtables. Did the rest perceive the White family as superior? Or
perhaps their choice of the Brady Bunch said that the Huxtables'
upper-class lifestyle seemed out of reach to them. Compared with
that of the Huxtables, the Bradys' lifestyle represented a much more
mainstream, and attainable, version of the family.

In many ways, the race of the television family did not matter. All
of the teenage girls on these family programs were adorable, smart,
or at least well-dressed, and nonthreatening to their brothers and fathers. They also adhered to an unspoken moral code. They dated boys
but did not indulge in sex. Most important of all, they did not have
babies. Occasionally a seemingly serious problem arose, like taking
drugs, for instance. But generally such problems were handled in a
show in which the parents helped the children resolve their problems
quickly.[10]

Reproducing Gender and Class
in the Family

The major difference between the Huxtables and the Bradys has to
do with the parents' identity. The Brady mother was a charming and
warm housewife who projected the image of a woman cared for and

protected by her good husband: Jessie Bernard's model of the provider.[11] In essence, hers was a nonthreatening image of motherhood. Terry and Dana may be less comfortable with Clare Huxtable, a successful lawyer with a strong personality. Perhaps this type of woman reminds them of the unpopular and masculinized stereotype of the assertive, independent, and hard-working Black woman who did not take any "crap" from her children or husband.

In the Brady Bunch family, Dad is the only breadwinner. That fact is likely important to the teen mothers. To eighteen-year-old Terry, who had lived with a single mother on welfare aid most of her young life, two-parent families lead wonderful lives. Although there may be family squabbling and bickering, when compared with her own life, these families are happy. In fact, in this show family quarreling seems healthy. Unlike Terry, the Brady Bunch teenagers have good relationships that withstand even skirmishes with their father. Terry thought about the meaning of the television show again: "I thought about the fact of not having a constant family life. I won't tell my son now, because if he asks any questions 'bout his father, I don't have any answers for him." Terry compared her situation with that of the Brady Bunch family and found it lacking. There was no legacy of strong family bond as demonstrated by the Brady father and son for Terry to pass on to her son. As her mother may have felt about Terry's questions, she dreaded the day her son would begin asking about his father.

The other meaning Terry attached to the Brady Bunch's family image came from the reconstructed nature of the family: two single-parent families, each with three children, living as one. This meaning tells us a great deal about Terry and Dana. Both teen mothers hoped for the possibility of a reconstructed family in their own lives. Equally important, Terry and Dana saw the image of a merged family, with a loving stepfather who cared for all the children, not just his own, as the kind of family and stability they wanted. Terry was, after all, the one who emphasized a father's responsibility to his children in her expectations of fathers. The Brady Bunch held out this hope.

Father as Status Provider and Protector

Despite their denials about needing fathers, the model of the father that Terry and Dana were articulating was one who could provide them with status and protection. Sociologists often assume that only middle-class women, like Diane Harris, receive a place in society through the transmission of their father's status. We tend not to believe that poor children receive either status or protection from their fathers. But while unemployed or low-income fathers may have some difficulty filling the provider role, there is evidence that they do bring a sense of status and protection to their children.[12] The father's ability to give his child status may come from more than being a good provider. The father's status may be just as important to low-income daughters like Terry as to middle-class daughters like Diane for knowing who they are and where and how they are expected to take part in the world.

When fathers are involved in their daughters' lives, the mothers do not have to take on all the responsibility for raising their daughters and the daughters do not require their mothers to do so. In effect, fathers bring balance to the daughter-mother relationship because their presence ensures that someone else will share in providing emotional nurturing to the daughter and mother, which takes on tremendous importance if the family is faced with a critical event like teenage pregnancy. Even if the family does not experience that kind of dramatic event, the father's treatment of the mother helps his daughter see that her mother, another woman, is someone special and a person with wishes and plans for the future. Further, during the adolescent years an alliance needs to be forged between parents to act on behalf of the adolescent or to mediate between the adolescent and the other parent. If the adolescent is a Black girl, the alliance between mother and father may be imperative if she becomes involved with her peer group or in sexual relations with boys, or when she confronts racist and sexist practices. In fact, it is precisely because Terry faced so many difficulties that she needed to have a father or someone acting as a symbol of authority in her life.

For the teenage girl, having a father in the home as a symbol of authority may be vitally important. The father may determine the relationship she has with teenage boys who come to visit her. Male authority is greatly respected by the male culture. The father has a powerful effect on how far young men attempt to go with his daughter. According to Elizah Anderson, "Upon encountering each other, both know something, that is, they know that each has a position to defend. The young boy knows in advance of a pregnancy that he will have to answer to the girl's father and the family unit more generally."[13]

At issue here, Anderson points out, is male turf right, a principle that the teenage boy and the father of the girl intuitively understand (Terry's father's visit could be interpreted as his way of establishing authority, although he was a little too late). As Anderson puts it, a boy may feel frustration because he must balance his desire to run his game against his fear of the girl's father. Yet these young men can often identify with the fathers of these young girls, since they may wonder how they might behave if they were in a similar situation.[14]

If Anderson is right, Susan Carter was very insightful when she claimed that her father, whom she perceived to be more powerful than her mother, may have been able to intervene in her relationship with Joney and perhaps prevented her pregnancy. But what I took away from Anderson's observations and my own is that it is not necessarily the gender of the person in authority that counts; rather, mothers who have authority may also be able to defend the family unit. For example, several adult mothers tried to control their daughters' sexuality by keeping check on their menstrual cycle and withholding information about sex and birth control. Their efforts were defeated, however, by forces outside of their family unit. The strongest such force was the ideology holding that women are unable to control their children. The problem for these teen mothers is not that fathers are the only ones who can act as authority figures or provide the protection and support that Anderson believes only men can do. More to the point is that in this patriarchal society, male authority is the only kind of power that is respected outside the family domain. Years ago, until so much went wrong, the old neighborhood women did not give in to that ideology. They had the kind of authority in the community that boys and girls alike did not challenge. Given another life situation, Lois Patterson might have felt comfortable with that kind of tough authority.

The Preference for Male Love

What other issues lie behind the search for father, the creation of a fantasy father, and the deep emotional feelings the teen mothers dared not reveal? The answers came during the end of a long interview with Terry and Dana when I asked them to tell me if they gained anything from being mothers. I thought that they might describe how much they enjoyed watching their children grow and learn—the kind of statements made by other mothers. Terry, who responded before Dana could, had a different view:

I feel like I get life from my child 'cause he gives me a reason to keep going and to strive for more so that I cannot only have more for myself but for him. Because when I think of just going on for me and I go, well, it's just me. But the thought that he's there too, is what really gives me that push to do more for myself. He's a good boy. He's saved my life in a lot of ways.

—In what ways?

He's slowed me down a lot from a lifestyle that I [would have] more than likely taken on if I didn't have him. When I've gotten discouraged and said, "Oh, what the hell, why keep dealing with that," I've always gone back to him.

Dana, easily caught up in the discussion, for once waited until Terry finished talking before offering her opinion:

He gives me a push, makes me strive to do better. Would I work? Would I be a bum? Would I be a street person? And he makes me think positive. Things that I want him to have, things that he wants me to have, I want to be able to give him. So, like Terry said, he's been very positive in my life.

—So he gives you a push and a shove. Would you say that's a kind of love you're not getting from your mother?

Terry answered before Dana could:

I got a lot of love from my mother. Put it this way, he gives me a lot of love that I'm not use to having from a male.

—Okay. Please explain to me what you mean.

Again, Terry was the first to answer:

I've never had a man, a male—I don't care if he's a baby or anything—love me, care for me. He does that. Although we get on each other's nerves, it's just that, maybe it's male love that I miss.

—So you think that there's something special about that kind of love. If he was a girl child, it wouldn't be the same.

No. It wouldn't. I don't know. I just love boys.[15]

Terry just loved boys, indeed. She transferred those feelings about male love onto her son, someone she saw as an emotional rescuer: someone who made up for all the love her father and other men did not give her. Dana giggled nervously, but she agreed. The deep emotional need expressed in Terry's and Dana's words took us into uncharted waters. Male love, after all, was the subtext of their stories. Terry added, "Everything my son achieves is going to be for me."

The two mothers' quotes certainly describe male love as being different in quality from female love, and male love was a powerful tonic to them. Perhaps it had more potency, magnetism, and authority for them than female love.

In Terry's comments about male love she expressed the desire to make her son's love central in achieving an experience different in texture from the female love surrounding her and familiar to her. That familiarity may have caused her to place more importance on male love and less importance on the female love she received from a support group of women (including her mother), which she implied was too woman-centered. She did praise her mother and cousins, but when she described the ideal mother she wanted to emulate, she talked about Mrs. Brady. Perhaps she saw her mother as a less appropriate role model because she was too old and too poor. Or as De Vonya said so ruefully about her mother at one point, she was too tired to serve as any kind of model for the daughter who needed love. Sadly, De Vonya's mother supported this view by presenting herself as a model of "what not to be." Perhaps Mrs. Brady was more suitable a model to Terry and Dana than their mothers precisely because of her status as the nonworking housewife of a powerful male.

Father Loss

Talk of emotional loss resonated throughout Terry's interview: she lost her father early in her life, she found him and then lost him again, she wanted male love and then found a substitute in her son. *The American Heritage Dictionary* defines loss in three ways: the act of losing something, someone who is lost, and, in language that connotes an emotional affect, the harm suffered by losing or being lost. The concept of the absent father, which most sociologists use in describing fathers who are not available emotionally or financially for their children, does not sufficiently convey the emotional impact of that absence on children, in this case their daughters. Father loss is a more useful and powerful concept than mere father absence, because it conveys the depth of the emotional feelings of the daughters. If young women are more susceptible to pregnancy if they have experienced an acute sense of interpersonal loss (as Warren Miller's study of the psychological vulnerability that leads to unwanted pregnancy points out), father loss is a more useful term because it conveys a greater sense of that painful emotion.[16]

Terry's strategy for dealing with the loss of significant men in her life was to reshape her feelings: "I feel it's pretty bad when my son has to ask for his father. Then I also feel it's not my loss. It's the father's loss. He's losing out." Her words seemed to disavow her own feelings. She wanted to appear in control. To do so, in the next breath, she shifted the focus of attention away from herself onto her commitment to motherhood and to her son: "I enjoy kids. That's what I keep tellin' you. I think it opened up a lot of parts of me that I didn't know were within me. Before my son was born, I didn't know I was tolerant or had so much patience as I have. But I just enjoy him." However, she enjoyed the idea of motherhood more than the actual experience of it. Most of her discussion of male love and the joy of motherhood centered on her own needs. As she interacted with her son, her behavior spoke more of the images of motherhood than the reality: she criticized Cecil harshly, yelling at him several times when he interrupted us, ignoring him when he asked her questions. Terry's attitude toward her son is not surprising; after all, no matter how mature she tried to sound when she talked about her experiences, and no matter how often she professed to being a "regular old lady," she was hardly past childhood herself.

Being a "regular old lady" seemed hard for this mother and for many of the teenage mothers as well. Other mothers took to it more easily. Dana managed to play with both children, feed them, and keep up with our discussion, all at the same time.

The Lure of Motherhood

The teenage mothers certainly raised new questions about what was at the root of their desires to have babies. How did their ideas about motherhood relate to all I said about the men in their lives? Terry and Dana wanted the kind of male love they assumed men like Mr. Brady provided his family. Adding to that image was the happy, smiling Mrs. Brady, the image of a mother who received flowers, candy, and Mother's Day cards from the husband and children who unfailingly loved her. The teen mothers handled these images by trying to live out the traditionally accepted feminine role, focusing their attention on families and babies.

There is compelling evidence that the teen mothers willingly choose to have their babies as a way to meet their emotional needs. Their refusal to heed their mothers' and sometimes the babies' fathers' advice to have abortions or put the babies up for adoption demonstrates the powerful lure of motherhood.

When I would flip through popular Black women's magazines, such as *Essence,* so often prominently displayed on the teen mothers' bookshelves, coffee tables, or kitchen counters, I saw a few pictures of thin, shapely, sexy, and fashionable women writing about money, careers, marriage, and emotional commitment to men. Mostly I saw pictures of happy mothers with smiling babies nestled peacefully in their arms. These pictures are covert statements of a gender ideology that consistently, and almost perversely, socializes all girls in this society, regardless of race and class, to believe that the primary lifetime role for them is that of a mother.

It is not surprising, then, that the teen mothers saw motherhood as a way to meet their emotional needs. Motherhood did give the teen mothers a way of fulfilling both a social expectation and a personal desire. From the teen mothers' perspective, motherhood may be a resistance strategy: a way to gain control over their lives, as Terry's eloquent comments about her loss of the baby's father seemed to say. Having babies also enabled the teen mothers to engage in a fantasy of recovery; that is, they could make up for the loss of trust and lack of connectedness in their intimate relationships.

Unfortunately, this motherhood strategy is ill timed and does not work. Instead of giving teen mothers a way to deal with their circumstances and their despair, the strategy opens up a Pandora's box of problems and issues that, as adolescents, they do not know how to handle. As we shall see in the next two chapters, no one else knows how to handle them, either.

At issue in these discussions about motherhood is what C. Wright Mills calls "matters that transcend those local environments of the individuals and the range of [their] inner life."[17] In sum, these two chapters on the men in the lives of these teen mothers—their own fathers and the fathers of their babies—reflect the social situation of women's and men's relations in the wider society. We can see how these young women are shaped by external forces, especially by gender, race, social class, culture, and, to some degree, the media's depiction of mainstream families. The outer structure of these teen mothers' lives was such that their own cultural and practical arrangements of family life were supplanted by the notion that the Bradys' model of life was preferable to their own women-centered families.

Here we find yet another irony, in these stories replete with ironies. These teen mothers, who according to the popular view did not have good moral values, chose conventional and traditional family role models for their ideal family. This point will continue to be emphasized throughout this book.

Part Three

The Community's Response

Chapter Seven

Girl, Let Me Tell You about Welfare

I hear what they say 'bout me. "Yeah, she sits on her fat ass all day long looking at soap operas."

Seventeen-year-old Jackie Marley

On the day of her appointment with the welfare worker, Shana Leeds walked with me into the sprawling one-story building on Broadway and Fortieth Street in Oakland. She joined the line of people at the information desk waiting to receive a number. Although she had arrived early for her nine o'clock appointment, ten people were already ahead of her. At half past nine a brisk middle-aged Black woman directed Shana to a desk in a glass-enclosed office. Glancing at Shana's paperwork, the welfare worker explained that Shana's check would be delayed another week because she had not filled out her monthly forms correctly. We were ushered out of the office in minutes. This experience is typical for many teen mothers.

In 1990 over half of teenage mothers of age nineteen or younger were receiving welfare assistance.[1] An ongoing political debate concerns whether these Black teenage welfare mothers are victims of an uncaring society or have simply learned to take advantage of social policies. This debate colors the teen mothers' own views of themselves, and it affects their ways of dealing with the welfare process. The teen mothers develop various strategies to help them handle the stigma associated with welfare use.

Seventeen of the teen mothers in this study were on AFDC. Of the seven selected for in-depth interviews and observations, only two, Lois Patterson and Terry Parks, were long-term welfare recipients, as were their families. Most of the other teen mothers applied for welfare for reasons similar to Shana Leeds's: "My mother worked, but she told me maybe I should get on welfare. I needed help, and she can't give it 'cause she don't have any extra money for the baby." Like this teen mother, De Vonya Smalls also had no other recourse. Her mother's disability check was not enough to take care of her and her daughter, and she could not count on her father or the baby's father, because both were unemployed. De Vonya was determined not to stay on welfare for long, she said. Instead, she was planning to finish high school and find a job.

When I asked the teen mothers how they might support themselves without welfare aid, most saw only two alternatives to welfare: becoming prostitutes or selling drugs. Lois Patterson responded quickly and with great indignation to those alternatives: "There is no way in the world I would have to sell my body or sell drugs."

David Ellwood suggests that a woman who goes on welfare "immediately loses control of much of her life." Ellwood argues that administrators require information and verification: the welfare recipient should have virtually no assets. "If she reports those earnings, her check is reduced or eliminated. If she moves, she must report it. If she shares rent, she must report it. She uses food stamps at the market. She is labeled a 'welfare mother'—one of 'those welfare cheats.'"[2] For the destitute teen mother, choosing to become a welfare recipient rather than sell her body or drugs may be the best decision, but there are negative consequences even with this choice.

The Debate over Welfare Dependency

The AFDC welfare program was *not* designed as a support program for Black women and children. Originally the program, as part of the Social Security Act of 1935, was established to serve the needs of the "deserving poor," the needy over sixty-five years of age, the blind, and dependent children. At that time women were not expected to work, so it seemed reasonable to the Roosevelt administration that unfortunate women without men in the home should receive some kind of aid.[3]

After World War II, as more and more people became eligible to receive welfare, the program expanded. Population growth among children and the increasing number of widowed women heading families added to the swelling rolls of AFDC. As a result, most welfare recipients were poor women with children. In the turbulent 1960s, Black women began finding their way onto the welfare rolls. The 1960s growth in welfare spending was predicated on reformers' suggestions that some poor families, especially Black families headed by women, were in need of a family policy. But as I mentioned in Chapter 1, the Moynihan report turned that need into a negative assessment of such families. As Morris Janowitz puts it, "AFDC may be viewed as a response to economic and social pressures resulting from the rise of the single-parent family." But, Lar Levitan notes, the rules and regulations of AFDC operate to sustain the prejudices of the "respectable" elements of society.[4]

As Moynihan saw it, the low rate of marriage within the Black community, along with increasingly high rates of Black teenage girls giving birth, indicated that there was a breakdown in the Black community's moral structure, signaling that Black women were incapable of raising their children properly. The report concluded that the Black female-headed family had become involved in a "tangle of pathology."[5]

The Political Use of the Black Mother-Headed Family

The 1960s may have inspired conservative social control approaches like Moynihan's (although he was considered a proponent of liberal causes), but it was also a time when people attempted to advance their concerns for humanity. As a result of the Moynihan report, liberals began looking more closely at Black families, and they discovered that Black women lived in conditions quite different from those of White women. Liberals discovered two American systems of economy and families at work.[6] One system comprised mainly middle-class White women who nurtured their children in two-parent families (although there were also poor White women in this group). The other system

comprised mainly poor Black single mothers who were having a difficult time raising their children.

During the time Moynihan was publishing his report, people in the
Civil Rights movement and the Women's movement marched outside
the White House and through Washington, D.C., to show support for
the idea that Blacks and women should have equal parity with White
men. There were several attempts by liberals to seize the moment by
making welfare assistance more available to those in need. Liberals
believed that government had a moral obligation to give aid to poor
people. They argued that welfare use among Black women was the
result of structural forces emerging from their poverty and from the
racism that limited opportunities for Blacks.[7]

The liberals' position was that government is accountable for these
conditions and should give poor Blacks financial support to help them
against unemployment and racism, especially since Black women had
become part of the other America. Black women's poverty had become more permanent than that of White women; they tended to become involved in a welfare system that provided them with almost no
real training. Since Black women were unlikely to find employment
or eligible husbands, they stayed on welfare longer than White
women.[8]

Along the way, the Civil Rights movement changed its course, focusing on voter registration instead of on economic parity for Blacks.
To this way of thinking, the new voters' registration strategy would
bring Blacks to the voting booth, and through the political process
Blacks would eventually obtain more economic power. Thus, Black
leaders began to focus on developing elaborate voter registration
techniques. The Civil Rights movement missed the signs that voting
rights did not usually produce economic parity and that they should
place voters' rights alongside economic parity. Movement members
worked to defeat a bill that promoted government jobs for welfare recipients. At the same time, the Black community came under heavy
criticism by the general public for failing to provide moral leadership
to large numbers of Black single women with children who depended
on government handouts.[9]

Various attempts were made to make welfare a political issue.
Nonetheless, in the 1970s Black women's poverty grew worse. In ad-

dition, the percentage of poor families headed by women
along with the proportion of children who could expect lo
tional attainments, lower occupational status and income,
rates of early marriage.[10] Liberals were not able to overcome the political rhetoric of conservatives who convinced the general public of
the false claim that Black teenage mothers and welfare queens were
"ripping off" taxpayers.

Moynihan's report on the demoralized and disorganized Black female-headed family coincided with women's fight for the equal right
to earn a living—something that Black women have always had to do.
The Women's movement, comprised mainly of middle-class White
women, has put abortion rights and equal opportunity for women at
the top of its agenda. In the process it failed to account for racial and
class differences between its issues and those of Black women.[11]

Lacking the support of feminist and liberal political activists, many
Blacks came to accept the conservative perspective. There was a shift
in public political thinking in the Black community about who should
be held responsible for Black women's increased use of welfare. In
the 1960s and 1970s many in the Black community and among its
supporters blamed "the system" for the drugs and gangs invading their
neighborhoods. That view has been replaced by the one blaming
teenage mothers for the problems of the Black community.

Similar views were held by several social workers in Oakland and
Richmond who worked with the teen mothers. They expressed concern about "underclass types"—those who had babies to get welfare
assistance because they were too lazy to work. Why did poor teenagers
have children, if their only recourse was welfare? they asked me. The
only reason they could think of implied the moral unworthiness of
these teenagers. Not only did these children have babies, but they
also expected taxpayers to pay for the consequences of their deviance.
In the opinion of these social workers, such mothers reflected badly
on the rest of the Black community.

Some of the teen mothers voiced identical views about welfare
mothers. Diane Harris picked up on this common perception when
she said, in response to my questions about her attitude toward welfare mothers, "It's up to them. Some women figure, 'I can stay on welfare and get four hundred and seventy-four dollars,' or whatever else

they get. It's comfortable. I mean it's just too comfortable. They have
to want to get off." I asked her if people would say the same about
her. Adamantly responding "No!" Diane Harris made it clear she
planned to continue her education and marry some day, thereby distinguishing herself from those mothers whose long-term welfare assistance, she believed, was due to their personal character flaws.

Did these teen mothers conform to the popular assumption about
welfare mothers? The teen mothers knew all the stories about their
deviant characters, and they spent a considerable amount of time de-
fensively describing their lives on welfare.

Applying for Welfare

The teen mothers described how nervous they were at the thought of
going into the seedy and crowded welfare office: "I hated going down
there in the first place. It's like they look at you like, 'What you come
here for? [You want] money too?' They look at you with a dirty look
when you walk in the door and ask you every kind of question they
can think of." When I waited in line with Terry, I noticed many of the
workers, with no personal space to call their own, huddled over their
desks, hunched over typewriters, or talking on the telephone in full
view of everyone. (I wondered to what extent the workers' depressed
working conditions accounted for their rude treatment of the teen
mothers.) Some of the teen mothers who had heard these stories
about ill-tempered workers were so frightened that they asked friends
to accompany them to the welfare office. If a teen mother was not familiar with the procedure, the friend acted as a guide, informing her
of what to expect: "Me and my girlfriend went down. She told me,
'Go up to the window' . . ."

Even when a friend accompanied them, the teen mothers often
found the application process so mysterious that no amount of assistance clarified it for them. Evie Jenkins, displaying a talent for story-
telling, poked fun at the bureaucratic procedures and foul-ups:

And Welfare, girl: I went down there and honest to God, I could not believe
the things that went on down there. First of all, you go down, you take a
number. You wait. And if those people decide they want to eat cake while
they're waiting on you, they'll be eating cake and anything else they want.

And it takes nothing for them to remember to ask you how old you are and banging on a manual typewriter and then chewing and taking a bit of food and you're standing up there and then they'll ask you another question. It's awful. And so then they tell you to come back. "You should be here about six o'clock." And I said, "In the morning?" And she said, "Yeah."

I said, "Hell, I ain't camping out overnight." She said, "Well the guard is here and he gives out numbers." Honey, I got there at a quarter to eight. I was number twenty-seven. So therefore three hours later they told me they couldn't see me. I had to come back in the afternoon. I went back at twelve-thirty as they requested, and I didn't get seen until two-thirty. And I had a real nice social worker, but I felt some of the questions . . . I mean, your life is no longer your own. There is nothing private about it. They want to know everything except the amount of gold you got in your teeth. And if they think you can hock that and get it out of your mouth, they will ask you.

Evie's story may have been depressing, but at that moment we were laughing so hard that she had trouble finishing it.

Lois Patterson's descriptions of her welfare experiences veered between being funny and sad as she talked about the slow procedure. She waited in long lines for an application, waited to find out if the application was accepted, waited to hear from the social worker, and then waited for information on a lost check:

Welfare—you've got to run down there at least once a month or twice out of the two months. Somebody done mixed up some kind of paper or this is cut off because you haven't put a paper in. But you know the paper's there. I haven't gotten my health care card. But it's in the office. I know that's what it is. And I haven't called her.

The welfare office called and asked me to call them at 8:30 this morning. I called her. She wasn't in and hasn't called me back yet. Now I went and applied on June 12 and I was suppose to get a check on the twenty-seventh. Both of my checks got lost, and I have to wait. I get forty-three dollars in food stamps a month. That's all. People think you're living in high class on welfare.

Lois found the treatment "degrading":

They cut me off welfare for three months. Because I didn't sign a date in on my monthly forms. Yeah, they cut me off. Why did it take three months to get back on, to call me? I asked them. "Don't rush me," the worker told me. I said, "Okay, I m going to call your supervisor." I got her and they still didn't send it. I went over to her supervisor. That's when they gave me the first hundred dollars.

—What did they say to you?

They told me, "Oh, you'll get the rest."

   Waiting in line or waiting for the rest of the check were difficulties
shared by Lois and Evie, who had very different family backgrounds
and welfare histories. Such problems were also shared by most of the
welfare mothers in this study. In a way, these interviews describe
teenage mothers caught up in struggles over form and image. First,
they have to struggle against a stiff and cumbersome bureaucracy that
often ignores them or, if they do not follow the rules or if the workers
do not like them, treats them with contempt or slows down the paperwork.[12] Second, once these teenagers became involved in the welfare system, they had to struggle with a pervasive and demoralizing
image of themselves as welfare mothers and cheats—in exchange for
the monthly stipend.

The Welfare Baby

Terry Parks was nine years old when she heard a neighbor call her a
"welfare baby." A few years later, Terry realized, "A lot of people make
fun of people on welfare." She became increasingly embarrassed
about being labeled a welfare baby. In Terry's mind, the label made
her seem different from a nonwelfare baby in ways she felt but could
not understand. When I pressed her to explain those feelings, she did
not do so directly but instead focused on the nonwelfare status of a
girl she knew as a way to describe the impact of the welfare label on
her dignity:

I know this girl who stays a couple of blocks down the street from me. She
don't like being considered on welfare. It sounds . . . (laughs). I mean, [lis-
ten] to the way it sounds: "Welfare." That's it. It just sounds so bad. Her father and boyfriend, them's the type that give her anything she wants and she
has a boyfriend who gives her money and spends all his time with her and
stuff like that. So welfare would be like puttin' her down. That's low to her.

I heard the envy in Terry's voice as she used the example of the girl
down the street to talk of how the label of being a welfare user lowered her status.

The result of this lowering of status, Terry made clear, was a lowering of her self-esteem. She also contrasted her feelings of being considered a welfare baby with the good feelings she had during the brief time she was not on welfare. She recalled how excited she was when her mother joined the army. For a brief period, Terry said, "We lived like normal" families. Just three years later, a pregnant Terry filled out her own application for welfare assistance.

I asked her if people made fun of her now. She did not have any of those old problems, she said: "Nobody knows. You know, it's not like I expose it just generally. I don't want to hear people say 'You're getting your welfare check today.'"

As a group, the teen mothers believed that the ostracism and contempt started in the welfare office, when they went through the application procedure and had to confront the workers' demeaning attitudes. This demeaning process, which began in the welfare office, continued in their own community. The teen mothers pointed to the many neighbors and friends who became hostile to them, stereotyping them as scheming, lazy, "welfare cheats," who used their bodies as baby-making machines for profit.

Twenty-one-year-old Irene Logan, who made her first trip to the welfare office at eighteen and went again when her marriage broke up, also articulated the subtle blows to her dignity and self-image:

Other people's reaction to me was the worst. When you're standing in line to buy groceries and the looks of other people staring at you (draws out the words). When you have food stamps and pay for your groceries or when you're cashing a check. It would be a really big hassle. "Is this check stolen?" "Is this your check?"

It was a trip. Other people judging you without them even knowing how you feel as an individual. Oh, you have no rights. You have no rights to dress nice or want something out of life. Who are you to want this?

People who believe the stereotype of these young mothers do not consider how these mothers, many of whom are just beginning their adolescent years, feel about such constant assaults on them, and how hard many of them work to overcome the negative labeling of them.

Joseph Rogers points to labeling as the "essential component of social order." According to Rogers, the labeling of others is a way people make meaning out of a complex society. But the resulting "stamp of a stigma," he warns, can have devastating consequences for those who are labeled. Rogers writes, "An integral part of labeling consists of a divisive strain serving to divide groups into heroes and villains, believers and infidels" or some other "dramatization of virtue." According to Rogers, epithets, in this case "welfare cheats," are not "mere figments of the sociological imagination." As weapons in the hands of powerful people, labels are capable of inflicting injury, "since they serve to define, demand, and even destroy." These terms of degradation could result in ostracism.[13]

The "welfare cheat" label has the power to control and to "hurt deeply and long," as Rogers puts it.[14] It made Terry feel "low," creating what she experienced as a class separation between her and the nonlabeled girl who lived down the street. Lois Patterson felt its sting in her landlords' attempts at separating welfare and nonwelfare mothers into two class categories. Diane Harris's attempt to separate herself from other welfare mothers also demonstrates the power of the welfare label. Shana Leeds and De Vonya Smalls both made it a point to say it was their mothers who insisted they apply for welfare. Evie Jenkins made sure to say several times that she had gotten off of welfare. Susan Carter, who failed to qualify for welfare benefits because of her mother's income, said she was glad not be on welfare: "It's too embarrassing."

The Sex Question

The worst part of applying for AFDC—the one that made the teen mothers agonize, the one that invaded their privacy—was the requirement that they answer questions about their sex lives. Some of the teen mothers were still visibly upset as they described their embarrassment. Shana Leeds remembered filling out the application: "They asked when I had sex, where I had sex, and how often." Feisty Lois Patterson refused to answer the questions: "They get personal, but I tell them, 'I don't know.'" The rest of the teen mothers believed that if they did not answer the questions about their sexual relations, their application would be turned down. Evie Jenkins said, "When you get down to that office and wait around, they will ask you everything about sexual intercourse and how you got that child. They want to know when you did it, how you did it, how many times you did it." De Vonya Smalls tried to avoid answering the questions: "They ask,

'How many times you had sex with your man?' I said, 'I don't know.'
And they said, 'Oh, yes you do. You know.'"

Why is it so important to the interviewer that De Vonya "know"?
The official position is that the state wants proof that the teen mothers are actually involved with the men they claim were the babies' fathers. Since the young mothers each had to obtain a court order for
child support after filling out the AFDC application, it was necessary
to establish paternity. The Child Support Enforcement Act of 1975
was created for just such a purpose: it was intended to require women,
like De Vonya Smalls, to cooperate in establishing paternity and locating the absent father before they could collect child support.[15]

Though the sex questions may be a required part of the bureaucratic procedure, I am also aware that the people involved with the
teen mothers—social workers, teen counselors, church members, and
even De Vonya's interviewer—seemed to be preoccupied for one reason
or another with the sexual lives of the teen mothers (that was not the
way I saw it when I set out to interview the teen mothers). Beyond the
bureaucratic rationale, this information is psychologically useful to
the workers involved. Some of the questioning persons—social workers, school teachers, or Alternative Center counselors—compared her
or his own moral behavior with that of the teenage mother being questioned. The teenage mothers' sexual life seemed to fascinate these in-
quiring minds—a phenomenon all too common in sexually repressed
societies. As Goffman writes about stigmatized people, "Should the
stigmatized person fail to present [her] failing, the normal may assume
the task."[16] Teen mothers' admissions of sexual relations with the men
they claim are involved with them is a way for these people to "peg"
these mothers—to confirm, in their eyes, their assumptions about
them.

Obtaining Child Support

After they answered the sex questions, the teen mothers had to hope
that the babies' fathers would cooperate with them. Instead, seven of
the teen mothers said that to their astonishment, when the men made
their court appearances they denied being the babies' fathers. The
judge had to order them to take blood tests. The teen mothers were
able to prove the fathers' paternities and win the child support, but to

no avail. All seven fathers told the court that they were unemployed and could not pay child support.

Lois Patterson was able to collect child support from Ronald, her baby's father. She had hoped to use the child support money to pay for child care so that she could look for work and get off of welfare. While she succeeded in making Ronald pay her child support, she lost more than she gained. The father's child care support reduced her welfare benefits by the same amount, and to make matters worse, the baby's father, angry at her having the court make him pay child support, stopped his weekly visits to his son. After all the "hassles," as she put it, "I'm still on welfare." Eighteen of the mothers did not bother reporting their babies' fathers for child support. Five of these mothers refused to list the name of the father on their babies' birth certificates. They wanted to have nothing else to do with the men who treated them so badly.

The Cost and Benefits of AFDC

Were they getting a free ride as taxpayers think? Lois Patterson did not think she was getting anything free when she received only half of her monthly check, nor did she think so when the monthly check came late. De Vonya Smalls did not think so when she found it difficult to pay the rent on her apartment in the Acorn housing complex with her welfare check. Terry Parks and Dana Little did not see themselves as freeloaders either, since they were afraid of losing their apartment because of rigid welfare policies.

Most of the teen mothers were unable to pay household expenses out of their monthly $498 welfare checks. Terry showed me her monthly budget, based on a $498 monthly AFDC income, which usually fell short of her family's needs:

$250	Share of rent for two-bedroom apartment
50	Share of utilities
115	Share of food (she did not receive food stamps)
14	Laundry and cleaning
20	Milk and children's medicines
10	Transportation
29	Clothing, diapers, and unexpected expenses
$488	

Often, when she fell short of money before the next welfare check was due, she bought less food for her family. She cooked many "potato meals" for them because potatoes were cheap and filling.

Occasionally, by buying less food or not going to the laundry for a week, she managed on her budget allowance until the next check arrived. More often, however, Cecil needed something unforeseen before the end of the month (when according to her budget she should have ten dollars left over). She would have to borrow money from Dana, or Dana would have to borrow money from her.

I asked the two mothers and other teen mothers if they would receive more money if they had additional children. Most of the teen mothers did not think so. Others were vague; they did not know what extra benefits they would receive for the second child. Terry and Dana thought they could receive fifty or sixty dollars more a month, but they did not think the extra money could support a second baby.[17]

While most of the teen mothers were critical of the welfare system, a few admitted that they saw welfare assistance as a blessing. It meant they could set up their own households or stay at home with their children. Three out of four teen mothers cited child care problems as another reason to stay on the program. They did not mention reliance on their mothers or their extended families for child care. Lois Patterson referred to the old model of adult mothers devoted to helping with grandchildren. She compared that model with the new youthful and active grandmothers who could not or would not help: "See, mothers have changed. Grandmothers are going out and having fun, and they're not babysitting. Not, like, I was fifteen when I had my son. My grandmother took care of him. But the tendency for parents to take over is gone. These women are working." Some teen mothers said they could not count on their mothers' help because, "On Monday she might be available, and on Tuesday she might not be." One teen mother refused to ask her mother for help with child care because she felt guilty that she could not afford to pay her for babysitting. Other teen mothers did not want to ask their mothers for help with child care because, like Evie Jenkins and Shana Leeds and their mothers, they fought over control of the child.

The most important welfare benefit in the teen mothers' eyes— more important than being able to stay home with their babies—was health care. Terry put it this way: "The only thing that's good that comes out of AFDC [is] because I have to take Cecil to the doctor every month." Most of these teen mothers shared Terry's awareness that she would not be able to find a job offering adequate health care benefits. For that reason alone, she said, she could endure the ugly words and rude treatment by others.

The Temporary Use of Welfare

Despite the stereotype of these teen mothers as freeloaders, and despite their own acknowledged need for health care and the ability to stay home with their children, all of them said they believed that working for a living was better than receiving welfare. All the teen mothers stressed a strong work ethic when we talked about welfare. I suspected they used their work ethic as a way to overcome the welfare stigma. As Roleta Mimms said, "My mother told me something like this: 'If you don't need it, you shouldn't get it. Teenagers shouldn't want to be on welfare. They ought to really go out and look for them a job.' 'Cause, my mother said, 'if you work, then that'll be more money and it would be better for [you] and [your] child.'"

Terry Parks, who had been on welfare most of her life, recalled receiving a similar warning from her mother: "My mother told me that she didn't want me on it a long time like her. She'd rather me work a little bit. She just says it's not good income." Before De Vonya Smalls's parents became disabled, they had worked hard most of their lives. Mary Smalls told me that both of them wanted life to be better for De Vonya. They "just knew," De Vonya said, that she would work. When she became pregnant, her mother suggested she apply for welfare but added a warning: "Welfare is temporary. It is not to be abused." In her mother's thinking, people who had to receive AFDC on a permanent basis were truly desperate types.

The Cautionary Tales Strategies

The teen mothers told me that their mothers often gave them motivational speeches about the personal work habits they thought would help their daughters. De Vonya said of her mother, "She was always telling me, 'You need to get along with people, get to work on time, and promote yourself. Just be willing to do what is necessary to get a job.'" But De Vonya was not as optimistic about her future. She spoke of her future in much the same way Susan Carter did when she criticized her mother's work as too demanding and low-paying. De Vonya's view was influenced by the cautionary tales of friends who did not find work: "It's hard to get experience unless you go to a training school. I have a girlfriend who went for accounting, but she just tried [to find a job] and they said, 'That wasn't enough.' She still needed experience." De Vonya lamented, "It's hard. It's hard."

Some teen mothers reported that they did try to find work, often at Nation's and McDonald's (or Mickey D's, as they called the fast-food chain). Older women, like Evie Jenkins, who had worked at some point, spoke proudly about their work history. Their interviews revealed a common pattern among welfare recipients that is noted by sociologists: most used AFDC for support during the baby's early years and again when they confronted a crisis such as a job loss or health problems. For example, Mary Jo Bane and David Ellwood and others show that most welfare recipients use public assistance as a temporary support, and abandon it as soon as circumstances permit.[18] Frank Furstenberg Jr., who examined the experiences of three hundred Black women who gave birth as adolescents, found the same pattern of AFDC use as a temporary solution only. He found that among the women in his study, chronic or near-chronic welfare dependency was the exception rather than the rule.[19] This pattern runs counter to the conservative ideology about welfare mothers.

The Welfare Mom: Lois Patterson

Relational issues are also important in understanding the teen mothers' welfare experiences. Furstenberg's study also finds that some teenage mothers with limited social support are at higher risk of becoming dependent on welfare than those who have strong social support and educational backgrounds.[20] Lois Patterson's description of her life contrasts sharply with that of Evie or De Vonya. Lois, a twenty-seven-year-old mother of two children, had been on welfare most of her life. Every month, "if it arrives on time," she received six hundred dollars from AFDC and forty-three dollars in food stamps. When I met Lois, she was sharing a ramshackle two-story house in East Oakland with two children, two sisters, their two children, and her elderly grandparents. The tree-lined neighborhood seemed nice enough, but according to Lois, at night the street turned into a "drugger's paradise" and she often watched drug deals taking place.

Lois, a tall, heavyset, chain-smoking woman, looked older than her age. She swayed when she walked into the living room for our first visit. I caught the smell of alcohol on her breath as she sat down next to me. Lois's life had been turbulent. Her father left the family when she was three. One day, a few years later, her mother "went to the store" and did not come back: "She just ran off and left. My daddy left first and then my mother. And we didn't see her again." Lois remembered waiting until dark for her mother to return from the store. Finally, her eldest sister ventured outside to call their grandmother from the corner telephone box. Lois's grandmother arrived a short time later in shock and in tears: "My grandmother decided to move into this house, and take care of me and my two sisters. And we've been livin' here ever since."

Lois's two children have different fathers. Her first child, Ronnie, was born shortly after her fifteenth birthday. Lois received AFDC allotments and child support for him, although it took her a long battle to collect that child support. When she talked about Geraldine's, her second child's, father, Lois conceded that her luck with men was "all bad." She had high hopes for what she thought was a good relationship, but he dropped out of sight when she was four months pregnant.

Lois was anxious to get away from her sisters and grandparents, whom she called "unsupportive" and "nosy." Whenever we talked about the baby's father, the family fights over money, or her desire to move away from her extended family, Lois would lean over to whisper her comments in my ear.

Lois had tried to move several times, but, "Who's going to rent to a welfare mother?" she asked. She was still waiting to hear something from the Oakland Housing Authority regarding her application for a Section 8 apartment she had applied for nine years earlier.

Lois Patterson's lack of education, little family support, and long-term use of welfare qualified her for that "high-risk" group cited by Furstenburg. She tried to find work, but each time she failed to pass the required test. She told me a story that was really a cautionary tale about what could happen to a person who has few adequate skills. She remembered the time she attended a job training program as part of the AFDC requirement. In the interviewing phase of the program, which she unfortunately did not pass, she was taught to be friendly during interviews and to compliment the interviewers on any personal items she might see in their offices:

I went to one interview and I use what they taught me. This woman said, "Don't be looking at the stuff on my desk. Might come in here and rip me off." I said, "Well, excuse me. You know, that's what they was tellin' us how to do."

They cut me off because I didn't go in anymore. And I told 'em, "I already went to that garbage." They're going to show you how to fill out an application, how to talk to people. It don't work.

Lois laughed nervously while telling me this story. She remembered swearing to herself after that incident: "I ain't never goin' on an interview no more."

I came away from Lois's house with two contradictory impressions of her reaction to the job interview. Some people would argue that she used this humiliating experience as a way to justify, in her own mind, staying on welfare. But it was also possible that she was deeply affected by the worker's harsh reaction to her failed attempt to be cordial. After all, her self-esteem was at stake in the interviewing process. Further, Lois did not have the skills necessary even for learning a new trade. She may have felt so stressed about her lack of qualifications that she used the job interview failure as a way to remove herself from the job training program. One counselor discussed other teen mothers' similar problems: "If you want to train to be a nurse, but you can't be a nurse unless you can read and write, then you can't even go through the training program. So that's where people like the ones you mention fail right there, because they don't even have the basic skills to try and complete the program." Aware of her lack of skills and of the inability of the job training program to train her, Lois may have felt hopeless about finding employment.

Welfare or Marriage

Welfare reduced the teen mothers' dependence on the labor market. Welfare also reduced the teen mothers' dependence on men for social support, but for some teen mothers the only way off welfare was through marriage. Roleta McMann, who had received AFDC for ten years, learned the trade "doing hair." When she did not earn enough money, she had to apply for welfare assistance again. A few years later she became ineligible for AFDC when she married. Before the year ended, she had separated from her husband and had to apply for AFDC again. As this example illustrates, teen mothers are caught in a catch-22. They could marry to get off welfare, but many of these marriages fail. More important than failed marriages, the shortage of eligible Black men makes it highly unlikely that Black women, even without children, will ever marry. If they do, they are likely to divorce soon and not remarry.[21] Both Evie Jenkins and Lenora Jones married and divorced their babies' fathers.

Welfare and Housing

In Chapter 3 I noted that the teen mothers spent a great deal of time working out housing arrangements. The Alternative Center expressed concern over the girls' housing problems, but so far other agencies had not followed suit. Whatever housing arrangements the teens made, the choice usually fell between "really bad" and "not too bad" housing.[22] At one of the housing projects I visited, the tenants erected a modest plaque marking the spot where five-year-old Anton Roberts died when he was caught in crossfire between gangs earlier that month. There was the weed-choked patch next to the apartment building where, in the morning sunlight, Evie Jenkins tended to her begonias and collard greens before the drug dealers came out at night. Seventeen-year-old Melania Lowan had to move from there: "My friend's apartment is only big enough for her family. She don't have much room, so I have to move. I can't get housing because I'm on welfare." This teen admitted, with a sly smile, that she gave me the interview because she thought I could help her find an apartment. If Melania could not find housing, she would have to sleep on the floor of a friend's or neighbor's home.

Melania Lowan and Lois Patterson lived in a neighborhood of tree-lined streets and old, single-family houses. Both teen mothers complained that they were afraid in this neighborhood. Lois had a name for her street: "This is Hubba street. The task force is on this street every day. Hey, some of these little punks were going to show my son Ronnie some little rocks. I went down there with a baseball bat. Those boys went runnin'. Now it's crazy. Like I said, I've got to get off this block." In fact, tough and streetwise Lois had become involved in a few street fights: "Hey, I wasn't going to let them little punks beat on me. I clobbered them," she beamed. Lately she had grown weary of the fights and the neighborhood. But she could not rent an apartment on her own because she was a welfare mother with two children. In other words, she felt that the stigma of being a welfare mother limited her reputation and mobility, as labels and stigmas do.

One afternoon I arrived at Lois's home to find her excitedly waving a letter from the Oakland Housing Authority at me. After a wait of nine years, she was finally going to move. We talked about the new apartment. I was apprehensive. It was located in an area tightly controlled by drug dealers. She assured me, "It's a lot better than the area I live in now, I bet. I've got to get off this street." If she did not take the apartment, the only alternative for her was an apartment in the Acorn houses, where De Vonya Smalls had recently moved (Acorn did not discriminate against welfare mothers). But Lois did not like the alternative: "I shore don't wanna move into no Acorn housing."

Face-Saving by Covering-Up Strategies

Teen mothers like Lois Patterson may not be able to hide their welfare status from landlords, but as Terry Parks mentioned earlier, they do have some control in their private lives over who knows about it. Terry was not the only one to hide her welfare status. Goffman's term "covering" best illustrates these strategies. According to Goffman, covering necessitates an attitude or pose that others (in this case, non-welfare mothers) will not find offensive. Laud Humphreys also used that concept to explain a similar phenomenon in the gay community.[23] Analyzing gays' attempts to handle negative labels and stigmas about themselves, Humphreys deduced that their imitation of heterosexual marriage, for example, was designed to elicit acceptance from the straight segments of society. Society may find homosexuals who profess fidelity in marriage to be less offensive than those manifesting promiscuity.

"People would be able to tell," was so overriding a fear among the teen mothers that they were ever watchful of others' perceptions of them, and they developed strategies to cover the "welfare cheat" image. Terry and the others told stories about striking a "pose," as Goffman would say, to handle the "put-downs."[24] What is missing from Stack's cultural strategies study is the involvement of the self in compensating for the loss of dignity, a concept of deep strategies that Goffman understood. These interviews reveal three types of impression management strategies: some put their efforts into dressing up their appearance as well as their emotional states (the deepest of strategies), others avoid being spotted at the welfare office or other locations that might give their status away, and others rewrite personal biographies in an effort to hide signs that might give them away.

Dressing Up

Teen mothers who were also welfare babies, like Terry, told of being encouraged by their mothers to "dress up." Since being on welfare was taken as a reflection of character traits, dressing up was considered a way to convince people that the teen mothers were like the "normals" who earned a living. Terry filled her stories about her family's years on welfare with remembrances about the tremendous effort her mother put into finding ways to make extra money so that she could buy "extra things like clothes" for her family to offset the welfare stigma:

And you always had to have the fashion things: your hair, and this and that. I mean, just [like] the working parents gave [their kids]. We had just about the same. When I was growing up, you really didn't want nobody to know that your parents were on welfare. People are always down on you when they think you're on welfare because they think you're lazy and you can't get a job. That's what the average person thinks.

—Have you seen people who look like they're on welfare?

Yeah. You can tell (laugh). I mean, you can tell because welfare just supplies you with basic needs. I think the way we grew up, we were always popular. I think if we had been real bummy or kinda [with]drawn kids, and dressed badly, people would be able to tell.

Why did Terry's mother expend so much time and effort, not to mention money, to make this impression? Terry wanted to avoid the "put-downs." "Now people can't tell if I'm on welfare," the teen mother informed me. Terry also dressed up her emotional feelings, recalling that as a young child she felt compelled to put on a "happy face" around people, striving to be popular among her friends so they would not think of her as poor and needy. Sometimes putting on a happy face meant that when Terry visited friends' homes and was invited to have a snack or dinner, she pretended she was "too stuffed" from eating earlier at home even though she was "dying to eat." All of Terry's efforts at managing the "happy face" were to convince her friends that her family had plenty of food.

Diane Harris also worked on putting on a happy face. "I don't hold myself like I'm poor. I am poor, but I don't carry myself like I'm poor. You can't get around being Black. You can't hide being a woman, but you can hide being poor. I don't wanna be poor. I'm not going to submit to being poor, and I'm not going to tell people I'm on AFDC. Some people know I am, but I'm not going to tell everybody." Obviously, being poor and being associated with the welfare mother stigma was very painful to Diane. Diane's statements "I don't hold myself like I'm poor" and "I'm not going to submit to being poor" suggest that she would use sheer will power to hide her poverty and rework her feelings, dressing them up to feel better about herself in order to make herself less vulnerable to the stigma associated with welfare mothers.

Diane talked about her experiences as we sat in her neat, well-furnished apartment, with its expensive furniture and framed posters mirroring middle-class comfort. This presentation of self and home revealed an impression management strategy on Diane's part that functioned in two ways. She dissociated herself from "those welfare types" by dressing up her emotional state to present herself "like I'm not poor," and that same need compelled her to dress up her home to make a public front so that others would not know the truth about her class status. In effect, Diane created a false "dressed" self to offset the false "deviant" self that others took as representing the real Diane Harris.

Avoiding Being Spotted

Some teen mothers said that whenever possible, they avoided being seen at any locations that might give clues to their real status. Lois Patterson was careful not to let friends catch her entering the welfare office. Shana Leeds refused to shop at the local grocery stores when she had to use food stamps—a good way for neighbors to find her out. When she lived with her mother, Terry Parks waited for her mother outside the supermarket when her mother was using food stamps.

Rearranging One's Biography

Some of the teen mothers' strategies were designed to serve two purposes: to hide their welfare status and their young ages. They did so by rearranging their personal biographies. Evie let everyone but those close to the family believe that she had gone away to attend high school in another state. (For three years after the baby was born, her mother Marie, who had her own strategy, refused to tell her friends that she was a grandmother.) Diane Harris believed that she needed to hide her illegitimate son from eligible suitors, so she thought of letting him live with his father. Terry Parks said that she let her neighbors think she was separated from her husband.

Other mothers also admitted adding a year or two onto their ages. Theresa Shimms told me that her mother, who had her first child at fifteen, also tried to hide that fact by adding three years to her age. Even today, Theresa said, everyone thought that her mother was older than her actual age. According to Theresa, those strategies seldom worked. No matter how hard Theresa tried to cover up her status as a teenage mother, she admitted, most people in her community assumed, when they saw her carrying her baby, that the baby belonged to her and that she was collecting AFDC allotments.

The teen mothers also used another strategy in their attempts to "dress up" and therefore control their images: during the interviews they juxtaposed their welfare experiences with their strong work ethics and work experiences. These stories reminded me of Arlie Hochschild's observations about emotion management: "Institutional rules run deep but so does the self that struggles with and against them. To manage feelings is to actively try to change a preexisting emotional state."[25] As Humphrey's gay community borrowed the heterosexual form of marriage to win acceptance from straights, the teen mothers attempted to manage information about themselves by stressing acceptable modes of behavior, thus diverting attention from more unacceptable traits in order to lessen the oppressive judgments made about them. This strategy of redirecting everyone's gaze was used by Diane, who went along with the popular view about the class values of teenage mothers in an effort to separate herself from the stigma associated with teenage welfare mothers.

At the beginning of this chapter, I touched on contradictory and disturbing perceptions about poverty, race, and women's status.[26] Liberals think teenage welfare mothers are victims of institutionalized racism, sexism, and class inequality. Conservatives push a disturbing de Tocquevillian perception of individualism in which welfare recipients are "ripping off" hardworking taxpayers, cunningly manipulating middle-class generosity by having babies in order to collect welfare checks. Unlike the liberals, who see teenage mothers as victims of oppression, these conservatives maintain that the young mothers are winning the war against racism, sexism, and poverty.

When Lois Patterson and the other teen mothers told me about their efforts to find work and about their welfare experiences, I did not see any winners. As Mark Robert Rank notes, "Existing on welfare is psychologically difficult."[27] What I saw was the failure of those involved in the welfare system to connect in any meaningful way with these teenage mothers. None of the teen mothers enjoyed being on welfare or had children to increase their welfare payments. Instead, they expressed deeply felt resentment about having to raise children with little money, with no child care, no alternative way to provide health care for their children, and no alternative to living in neighborhoods controlled by drug dealers. Instead of wishing for more children or more welfare aid, the teen mothers spend their time reshaping their images and worrying about their lives. What I saw was the failure of the teen mothers to establish relationships with their social workers or anyone else who would understand that they were, after all, teenage girls in need of compassion and understanding.

Chapter Eight

They Are Saying Terrible
Things about Us

People judge you. They look at you in a different way.
Sixteen-year-old Carmilla Hopkins

Now that we have viewed the teen mothers through the ethnographic lens and discussed the teen mothers' views of their relations with their mothers, their babies' fathers, and their fathers and of their problems with being on welfare, in this chapter we look at another support system and its influence on the lives of the teen mothers: the teen mothers' peer group meetings and their relationships with the staff at the Alternative Center. At the Alternative Center the teen mothers could meet with other teen mothers and staff counselors to discuss the pejorative remarks made about them, express their feelings about being treated like social outcasts, and learn mothering skills. That the teen mothers would turn to the people they met at the Alternative Center for support and guidance is a powerful indicator that their families had not been very supportive of them at a crucial time in their lives. By joining the Center, they were also taking control of their lives and recognizing their need for advice and adult mentors.

The staff at the Center, along with two groups of visitors—White middle-class mothers and school teachers who also attended the peer group meetings—were committed to helping the teen mothers. Yet these groups became what Goffman refers to in his book *Frame Analysis* as *bystanders:* those who constitute the participant's framework.[1] In subtle and not so subtle ways, perhaps unintentionally, their strong conservative ideas undermined their support.

The Alternative Center

The Center operated with a grant from the Salvation Army. Its program's major purpose, as the pamphlets announced in bold letters, was to keep the doors open for unwed mothers. Originally it served as a home for unwed mothers from White middle-class families. When Black families began moving into East Oakland, the Salvation Army disbanded the home. In 1983 the Center developed programs geared to a population that needed outreach support. Its programs included an alternative school, day care, self-esteem development, parenting skills training, and, if needed, personal counseling.

I mention the Center's history because the changes that occurred in its East Oakland neighborhood when more and more Black families, teenage mothers, and drug dealers moved in had an impact on the small staff of people who worked there and on the support they could offer teen mothers. The Center's experience is also important because it reflects some of the problems of working with poor Black teenage mothers. The Center's very inability to achieve its goals combined with the increasing demands placed on the staff by needy teen mothers affected their working relationships with these same mothers.

When I began working at the Center, the director and the chief administrators were White women who headed a staff of three Black women program coordinators. Because the drug scene in the community surrounding the large, dull gray building had grown worse in recent years, most of the White staff began to dread their work, fearing the drug pushers in the community. Additionally, although they were very committed to the programs, they felt frustrated and overwhelmed by the teen mothers' many severe problems.

By the time I finished my work at the Center, most of the White staff had left and it was being run by a predominantly Black staff. The Black staff also wanted to leave but felt that they would have difficulty finding other jobs to match their skills and expertise, a problem they attributed to racist White employers. Several Black women were promoted at the Center as a result of the turnover. The newly promoted women also feared the neighborhood, but for them the central issue was one of being disadvantaged while at the same time having to work with the disadvantaged. The staff worried, too, that the funding agency would reduce the Center's financial support or make it more difficult to acquire funds, because the Center was staffed mainly by Black women who served a predominantly Black teen mother population. They were intensely concerned about the increased school and housing problems that the teen mothers would experience if the programs were discontinued.

The Support Group

As part of their parenting skills training program at the Center, some teen mothers had to attend weekly three-hour meetings, which took place at different locations but were always attended by three staff members. Five of the seven teen mothers took part in these group meetings. The purpose of the meetings was twofold: to help the young women handle the stress and strain of being teenage mothers and to create a supportive environment in which they could freely talk about a wide range of problems.

In the peer group discussions, the teen mothers talked candidly about daily issues and concerns. When Jackie Marley talked about her boyfriend, problems at school, or the difficulty of getting welfare, the other mothers nodded their assent, almost in unison. As Georgia Minns, more articulate than the others, spoke about her feelings, some stared down at their desks or rocked their babies slowly in their arms. Others laughed in agreement. They could discuss their estrangement from their own mothers and from the babies' fathers. The counselors encouraged this interaction and took a nonactive role in the discussions.

At the first meeting I attended, I made a rather general statement, hoping to get their response: "Some people think that teenage mothers are acceptable in the Black community." Several of the teen mothers looked at me and smirked. Junie Grant, a fifteen-year-old teen mother, was the first to answer. She described the way people stared at her whenever she took the baby outside. Junie remembered an especially uncomfortable situation that occurred during a visit to her doctor's office for her daughter's checkup: "The other day I had to take her to the doctor, and this woman, this lady, she made me real mad. She said, 'That's not your baby!' She was a Black lady, and she's telling me that's not my baby. This was at Kaiser in Richmond. And she said, 'That girl's too young to have a baby.' And I heard her in the background, and I just didn't say anything." Marnie Martin summed up the attitude of most of the people she encountered: "They think you're going to have this baby and get on welfare and stay on welfare. And not go to school and watch the soaps all day. 'Cause they were saying on the Oprah Winfrey show, 'We're taxpayers, and you're getting all of our money.'" Marnie said that as soon as someone found out that she had a baby,

I would get looked at up and down like, "Oh, look at her," when I go out in public with the baby. I'll have people look at me like, "Isn't she young to have a baby?" When they find out how old I am, they freak out! They look at me a lot differently. Just the other day, I was at school and this guy I was talking to, and I mentioned my baby girl (voice up). And he said, "How old are you?" And I go, "Fifteen." And he said, "What! And you have a baby girl. Oh, man, you're crazy." And he went on and on and on. I couldn't believe it, you know? God, why didn't he mind his own business, you know?

She also remembered how much it hurt when she learned that her friends were gossiping about her: "The other day I found out that the one who's suppose to be my friend isn't one. Now, I think that if you're somebody's friend, you should keep your thoughts to yourself about the bad points you really don't like. And she was talking with another group of people and my name came up and she said, 'Well, I think it's a shame that she's having a baby at this age.'"

An intense discussion developed among the teen mothers about gossiping friends. A few of them worried about the effects of that kind of gossip on their children. Junie Grant, the fifteen-year-old teen mother quoted earlier, said, "It hurts me a little when they say something, especially around Andrea, 'cause I'm afraid that when Andrea gets older, she'll understand it when somebody's puttin' me down and think that, 'Well, they're puttin' me down too.' It's kinda hard thinking how Andrea is going to grow up. 'Well, my mom had me so young and all these people are saying terrible things.'"

Gossip as a Mechanism of Social Control

The teen mothers' gossiping friends reminded me of the old neighborhood women who used gossip as a way to control the sexual behavior of young girls in the community. But the teen mothers themselves gossiped. Perhaps it was a way of gaining control over their own "deviant" selves. Several teen mothers had been among those in the nonpregnant group who gossiped about pregnant friends: "I use to talk about this girl I know. She had a kid the year before me." Everyone giggled. Junie Grant admitted, as did other teen mothers, that after she gave birth to her baby at age fourteen, she began to single out other "really bad" teen mothers for gossip. She was selective, though: the subject of the gossip had to be younger and have more children. "This girl has two kids, and she's twelve," she said, placing the girl in the "really bad" category. By putting the mother with two children in the group considered "really bad," Junie Grant was able to view her situation as "not so bad," in the same way that Diane Harris separated the "ghetto mentality" type from her own "accidental" type.

Gossip was thus used by the teen mothers as a means of social control—that is, it enabled them to identify and label young women whom they considered deviant. The teen mothers put teenage girls into classes of deviants, labeling them "good," "not so bad," and "really bad." The "good" category was reserved for nonpregnant teenagers. The "not so bad" category included teen mothers of one child who had been receiving AFDC for no more than one year. Teen mothers who had two or more children or had been on AFDC for more than one year were categorized as "really bad."

Junie Grant also gossiped about other teen mothers' length of time on welfare. The person gossiped about had to be on welfare longer than the person doing the gossiping: "She's been on for years. She ain't never gonna get off welfare." I asked the teens whether someone else could say they were just like the women they sanctioned. All of them scoffed at this idea, insisting they were different from the subjects of their gossip: "At least I didn't go that far," one teen mother reminded me.

Age-inappropriate pregnancy and excessive welfare use were not acceptable to Junie Grant. But she was a teenage mother and on welfare herself. One way to handle this contradiction was to reproduce a moral structure in which she could gauge others and come out the winner.

These resulting categories of good, not so bad, and really bad gave the teens some sense of order and control over their lives—as Joseph Rogers notes, labels have power.[2] Gossiping about others also diminished these young mothers' own need for emotional support from their friends. Instead of confronting the gossiper and asking for support from "so-called" friends or the "good girl," teen mothers found another group to belong to.

Sometimes the teen mothers' gossip became a means of wish fulfillment. Junie Grant said about another teen mother: "She's got a good family and ain't got the kinds of problems as me." Terry Parks said the girl she knew who lived down the street did not need to receive AFDC because the baby's father "comes around and gives her his time or some money." Terry seemed to be saying, "If only I had what she has," as if to emphasize that she had been shortchanged.

It's Like You've Sinned

At one point, the teen mothers shifted from the topic of gossiping friends to a discussion about the church and the way church members treated them. Since religion and church membership is so important to the Black community, I expected both to play a large role in the teen mothers' lives and in their stand on abortion. Some teen mothers said they considered it morally wrong to have abortions—an idea that seems to come from the Black community's general religiosity, although several of the teen mothers did not consider themselves to be "very religious" (they attended church on the average of once a month). Lenora Jones stopped going to church services when she became pregnant because she was ashamed of her "big belly." When she did return to the church after her baby's birth, she expected that the church members would, as she put it, "forgive me." Instead she was singled out for criticism by the church members: "The members of my church told me, 'God's not gonna forgive you for gettin' pregnant.'"

This discussion became so animated that one teen mother, Irene Logan, had to raise her voice to be heard above the others: "It's the

Christian belief. I had to go to church and say that I was sorry. I had to beg forgiveness from the church and be restored to membership. If you commit what I did, what they call a 'sin,' you couldn't become a permanent member. They'd let you come to church. But they'd make sure you'd feel the shame. It's like you've sinned." The teen mothers saw this treatment by the church members as a way of separating them from the "good girls." In their minds, the church was as concerned with class and status as the secular community. Elizabeth Rauh Bethel studied a Black community in the South and found that both the community and the church are punitive in their treatment of unwed mothers. When the pregnant girl's condition became obvious, "they turned her out of the church until the baby was born. There was little to do but endure the pregnancy and wait for the baby to arrive, because the birth ended the girl's period of imposed isolation. The young mother's return to respectability began where her public shunning had first occurred, at church."[3]

According to Bethel, "When she [came] to church she had to get up and confess, and she sang this song. 'I Believe I'll Come Back Home. I Know I Done Wrong.'" Bethel's description of the southern churches' attitudes about pregnant teenagers was replicated in this study in the teenage mothers' descriptions of their experiences with their churches.

According to De Vonya, "The Jehovah Witnesses strongly believe in marriage. When Nadine got pregnant, she couldn't go there for a while." Shana Leeds believed that her church gave more credence to a middle-class teenage mother's pleas for forgiveness of her "accident" than the poor teenager who, they assumed, was morally deficient. Shana said these girls were shunned by church members: "Yeah, they keep them out. They kick them out."

The church members believed that teen pregnancy was not the real "sin"; being an unmarried mother was much more of a problem. Theresa Shimms, one of the few teen mothers who considered herself religious and was an active member of the church until she became pregnant, stopped attending church during her pregnancy because she worried that the church members would not treat her well because she was not married. She waited until the baby was a year old before returning to the church. But Theresa feared their reaction so much that she kept the baby's birth a secret from them. She used the example of another teenage mother to make her point:

> I didn't go back to church when I got pregnant because part of it was that if I went to church everybody's going to say, "Look at her." They're going to be just like my family was. And then I went to church and they didn't know about the baby. They didn't even know I had a baby. And I felt really good 'cause there was another girl there and she was also the favorite of the church. And she had a baby. She looked so depressed. There was no way I could let them know. What are they going to say to me? How are they going to treat me? I couldn't take this anymore. I used to go to church every Sunday. Now I'd rather sit at home.

Theresa was worried that the church would ask her, "Where's your husband?" Most of the teen mothers believed that the church would not have shunned them or asked them to confess their sins if they had been married. These teenage mothers suggest that the churches' attitude about teenage pregnancy is similar to conservatives' opinion that teenage motherhood emanates from low moral values.

As I pondered the teen mothers' comments about the churches' attitude toward them and put this attitude alongside the teen mothers' discussions about family and friends, it became apparent that the teen mothers were caught in a struggle between competing values: those of the churches, which restricted the support given to others, especially to those they considered to have low moral values, and those of the family. Perhaps the teen mothers should not have been surprised by their experiences. The ministers and church members shared the general conservative religious philosophy about traditional marriage and family. But the teenage mothers said they hoped for "unending" support from the church, maybe because of an idealism that they had learned from a religious philosophy promoting forgiveness and that resonated with their expectation of continued mothering from their adult mothers. The teen mothers were ultimately disappointed and hurt by church members' reactions. Consequently, they did not see their churches in the same way that Andrew Billingsley proposes in his book *Climbing Jacob's Ladder* when he applauds the "strong potential" of the Black church to help troubled Black families.[4]

The Counselors

"Sinful and shameful." Unfortunately, this popular view of teen mothers also resonated in the interviews with the counselors at the Alternative Center. This staff of middle-class Black women, in their late thirties and early forties, college educated and casually dressed, had grown up in conventional middle-class families in which their parents stressed mainstream values of work and family responsibility.

Most of the counselors tried coming to terms with the needs of the young mothers. I often had the impression, however, that they believed these teen mothers' values were different from their own. As I worked among the counselors and talked with them on a daily basis, I began to notice that they often peppered their discussions of the teen mothers with references to their own strongly held "old fashioned" values: the values their families and churches taught them about a girl's sexual behavior. The counselors seemed to use their values as a way of distancing themselves from the teen mothers. Nonetheless, they did seem committed to helping these young women, whom they called "clients."

The counselors disagreed among themselves about the causes of teen pregnancies. A few thought that the teen mothers wanted babies as a way to have someone who would love them. Some thought that the teen mothers' problems stemmed from their low morals. Others attributed sexual activity and early motherhood to individual choice. Still others echoed sentiments I often heard from people in the community; most teen mothers came from "dysfunctional families." A few counselors, such as Claudia Wilson, a heavyset woman with a warm, friendly smile, believed that racism played a major role in teenage pregnancy. But she focused on the idea that the daily encounters with racism made the teenage mothers have little or no self-esteem. The counselor who worked with the Richmond Teen Parent Program told me, "We all know that the key here is racism and self-esteem. We've come to that conclusion. They don't feel good about themselves." It was this belief more than any other factor that impelled Claudia Wilson to stay at the center.

Another counselor, Ann Getty, readily admitted that despite her training in child developmental issues, nothing in her life experiences properly prepared her for the problems these young mothers brought with them. She remembered when she began to work at the youth center and the period of adjustment she had to go through during which she learned to hold her opinions in check. She laughed when she recounted some of her earlier experiences: "Look, when I first started doing this, Elaine, I used to be doing, 'Ahhh.' I mean I constantly had my mouth open. But now, not anymore. They can tell me anything. I'm tough now." However, she went on to say, in spite of having worked several years at the youth center, she was still dismayed by the sight of "little girls who were barely past being babies having their own." Other counselors confessed that they saw the teen mothers as "little girls who were giving in to a desire to have dolls they could dress up."

In their personal counseling with the teen mothers, the counselors stressed the same values they had learned from their families. Ann Getty placed a strong emphasis on teaching the teen mothers self-development and on their need to be responsible for their future: "I tell them they have to build their own life so that they can take care of the future." Underlying Ann Getty's motivational speech was the notion of individual responsibility, the same idea de Tocqueville said dominated the American mind of the 1800s. When I asked her if she had any thoughts about why so many Black teenage mothers were becoming pregnant, she explained, "The bottom line is birth control here in the eighties." "Why don't they use birth control?" I asked her. "They just don't take responsibility. It's too easy not to realize the consequences. Some of them don't think. They're young." She dismissed the arguments I gave her about some teen mothers' health problems, the lack of sex education, and the misinformation about birth control that might prevent them from using it. In Ann Getty's view, the teen mothers were unthinking adolescents who selected the wrong boyfriends and passively followed the path of least resistance. In a tense voice she described the deep sense of helplessness she felt in dealing with these issues: "I find myself sometimes getting too emotional. It's real frustrating. I don't want to hear about another pregnant person. I went to a conference on teenage pregnancy, and I said, 'I don't want to hear anything' and that's weird because that's what we were going to talk about. But talk is cheap."

"Talk is cheap." Other counselors made similar remarks. They felt burned out and unable to do more than talk about these problems. Sometimes these feelings caused them to react less than professionally to the teen mothers. Pat Fields, a counselor for five years in the

Oakland area, remembered the day she angrily confronted a teen mother in the Center's hallway, screaming at her when she learned the teenager was pregnant for the second time: "How could you do this? It's stupid!" Pat Fields understood that she had lost her professional demeanor, that she felt so powerless in face of these problems that she took her frustrations out on the teen mother whom she had "worked so hard to help." After that incident, Pat Fields took stock of her attitude and did the emotional work needed to exert control over her feelings. "Now," Pat said, "I don't feel anything about you the second time if you have another baby." Still, Pat said, eyeing a group of teen mothers sitting at a table across the room, she warned all the teen mothers that they would lose her support if they became pregnant with a second child.

Marty Richards, a counselor in the Richmond school district, also had to deal with her own negative feelings about the teen mothers. She said she took a professional approach to her job, but she was more emotionally involved in this work than she admitted. More than the other counselors, she took a keen interest in the personal lives of the teen mothers she counseled. She also judged them harshly when they did something she found offensive:

See, I don't like to see dirty children. And this one client, we were going to take the baby to another lady to keep while the mother went to Martinez. She brought the baby out to the car and he was dirty. And he had never been dirty before. As a matter of fact, I always complimented her on how she kept his hair slicked to the sides. And she got into the car, I said, "Where are you going?" Push had come to shove and I went out and bought them something. I mean it's a reflection. You don't want your kids looking like that.

I asked Marty whether the child's dirty appearance signaled larger problems or perhaps the teen mother had had a bad day. "No. She had given the child a birthday party. That was fine, but I think that washing their clothes would have been a little high on her list too," she said. In these comments there were judgments not just about the mother's laziness but also about her underclass status. The comments add to my point that teenage motherhood is often seen as a class stigma.

Whatever their attitudes, most of the counselors did work very hard at controlling their emotional reactions to the young mothers. But for a variety of reasons, maintaining that control was very difficult for them. First, the major function of their job was to care for others. Second, the counselors brought to the job an awareness of the enormous problems in the community: they lived and worked in the community and passed the drug dealers and homeless on their way to and from work. Third, they also knew about the complex consequences of teenage pregnancy. If one considers as well the counselors' traditional views about teen mothers' values and anxiety over keeping their jobs, it is not hard to see why counselors like Ann Getty, Pat Fields, or Marty Richards felt helpless about the teen mothers' problems and often treated the girls with little more sensitivity than the church members, perhaps as a way of distancing themselves from problems they could not change (the same observation could be made of the reaction of others to the teen mothers).

At times, though, the counselors did understand the teen mothers. Often, during the peer group meetings when the teen mothers discussion turned to the problems of being a single parent, the counselors forgot the class and age differences between themselves and the teen mothers. Several times the older women felt so compelled to talk about their problems with boyfriends, husbands, and children that they joined the discussion. One counselor often had to remind the others that the meetings were supposed to focus on the teen mothers, not on the adults.

During these lively discussions, the class and age barriers between the counselors and the teen mothers lifted and relations became more egalitarian as everyone focused on problems common to most women. Although class divisions were apparent in the counselors' perceptions of the teen mothers, gender and race issues united them so that they could identify in some ways with the teen mothers.

The Teen Mothers as Peer Counselors

As peer counselors, the teen mothers were given the chance to act as representatives of the Center at various community functions where they shared their experiences with other teenagers and people interested in such issues. The counselors believed peer counseling to be a positive role for teen mothers because it gave them an opportunity to acquire the skills needed to answer personal questions, especially about their sexual behavior—the subject on everyone's minds. In addition it was hoped that the teen mothers could use their experiences to dissuade other teenagers from becoming pregnant.

These teen mothers were quite capable of consciously manipulating their world. Often the counselors would ask the teen mothers to tell visitors from the community about the problems they were having receiving support from the babies' fathers or from their own mothers. The visitors were often teachers or people from another teen mother program who would drop by the Center to learn more about the Center's efforts to help teen mothers. The teen mothers would agree to discuss these problems. But when these meetings took place, the mothers' description of their experiences varied depending on the audience.

The Concerned White Mothers

I attended the teen mothers' meetings with a number of groups of concerned community women. At these meetings each teen mother spoke vaguely, but positively, about her experiences: "No, it ain't too bad." "I manage okay with my baby and school work." Mostly the teen mothers presented their experiences in a positive light, especially when they were addressing adults and certainly if White adults were in the audience. For instance, instead of painting a dismal picture of herself, sixteen-year-old Carmilla Hopkins told one group of concerned White mothers, who were visiting the Center to "better understand why these girls have babies so young," that her life was moving smoothly along despite being a young single mother. The concerned mothers seemed astonished by the statement. She seemed smug and proud of herself. But Carmilla may have been saying to the counselors that she would determine how she portrayed her life to others.

I was often amazed at the way the teen mothers' presentation of self changed depending on their perceptions of me. Sometimes the teen mothers would tell me stories of how wonderful their lives were going. I did not always believe them, and I would tell them so by citing my own experiences, along with knowledge of their family lives, to counter their tendency to "dress up" their experiences. At that point the teen mothers would admit that their presentations of their lives did not quite fit with their realities.

The teen mothers needed this strategy of denial. Carmilla had few ways of dealing with being poor and had little chance of getting out of her present situation. This may be the case with the teen mothers in Dash's study who wanted to appear as if they were on top of their lives by being knowledgeable about birth control despite evidence to the contrary. In Carmilla's case the good life had to be invented, because the sixteen-year-old mother did not have answers for why her life had taken the turn it did, and yet she did not want to be considered a loser. This is why she responded so glibly to the concerned White mothers.

By the time I sat in on the support group meetings, the counselors had become extremely frustrated by the teen mothers' refusal to make a "personal problem presentation," to "tell it like it is" when they met with the concerned White mothers at community group sessions. During one meeting a counselor took me aside, deep lines etched across her face, to ask if I could convince the teen mothers to present a more realistic view of their lives. The counselors thought that the teen mothers were ashamed to discuss their problems or had developed a code of silence about "discussing private business" with outsiders.

According to Goffman's discussion of stigmatized people: "The issue is not that of managing tension generated during social contacts, but rather that of managing information about failing. To display or not to display; to tell or not to tell; to let on or not to let on; to lie or not to lie; and in each case, to whom, how, when, and where" to disclose discrediting information about the self.[5] The teen mothers' concealment of discreditable facts concerning their experiences as teenage mothers may have been their attempt to "pass" (in the words of one teen mother) as "a normal teenager." Carmilla purposely concealed information that she was failing in school and that the person she identified as the baby's father told all his friends that he was not the father, in an attempt to hide her identity as a "deviant teenage mother" by which people had come to know her.

It was also possible to read in their rejections of the counselors' requests the classic adolescent struggle with adult authority. Even further, perhaps the teen mothers saw the irony in the fact that the same adults who considered them deviants wanted to hear all the details, thus verifying that opinion of them.[6]

The Teachers

One afternoon a group of five Black and three White school teachers from the Oakland school district visited the Center. The teachers asked the counselors and the teen mothers to help them develop strategies to handle the growing population of teen mothers in their classrooms. Instead of giving the glowing accounts that they gave the concerned White mothers, these young mothers confused everyone by mixing positive and negative aspects of their school situation. One teen mother told the teachers: "I'm in school and doing okay." Another one said, "It's hard being a teen mother and a student."

The teachers were perplexed by the teen mothers' double messages. The spokesperson for the group, a matronly Black woman, began to chide the teen mothers. In a voice ringing with acrimony, she told them that their moral behavior went against her own upbringing: "I just can't understand why girls would become sexual and have babies at such a young age." The other teachers remained silent.

Although the stated goal was for the teachers to ask for the teens' help, perhaps the teachers felt compelled to remind the teen mothers about their failings. Goffman's concept of the "identity peg" helps explain the attitude conveyed by the teachers at these meetings. For him personal identity is the unique combination of life history items that become attached to the individual with the help of these pegs. According to Goffman, "Personal identity has to do with the assumption that the individual can be differentiated from all others and that around this means of differentiation a single continuous record of social facts can be attached, entangled, like candy floss, becoming then the sticky substance to which still other biographical facts can be attached." One's being a teen mother was used as an identity peg by others as a way of singling out the mothers' personal qualities of badness: "The person becomes reduced in our minds from a whole and usual person to a tainted, discounted one. Such an attribute is a stigma, especially when its discrediting effect is very extensive."[7]

The statements of wrongness that helped stigmatize the teen mothers as morally deficient also allowed the teachers to continue to see the teen mothers as persona non grata. The counselors did not come to the defense of the teen mothers. The counselors believed these teen mothers had to renegotiate their relationships with people, learning how to respond to negative criticism about their sexual behavior without becoming defensive. In fact, the teen mothers had come a "long way," Pat Fields informed me. When they entered the program, most of the teen mothers had an "attitude" and "cursed out" people like the school teachers (and the concerned White mothers). Eventually, Pat hoped, the teens would learn how to handle criticism effectively without the usual anger they expressed by offensive language. Until they could respond to comments by "insensitive people," Pat was grateful for the teen mothers' silence. But the teen mothers had demonstrated verve and tenacity by trying to exert control over the image they would display and by choosing when they wanted to "pass."

The counselors' views about self-determination, morals, values, and cleanliness stood in the way of their ability to counsel these young mothers. As far as the counselors were concerned, the teens involved were morally bad teen mothers and irresponsible fathers, a reinforcement of the age-old double standard based on gender. But the counselors, the concerned White mothers, and the teachers (like the average Americans in a national survey), did not translate the teen mothers' circumstances into larger questions about that double standard.[8]

For example, the counselors did not ask why mostly women attended these program meetings designed for both parents' participation. Nor did they ask if the teen mothers' friends who gossiped about them also gossiped about the teen fathers' sexual behavior and their young age. The Jehovah Witnesses did not act punitively toward the teen fathers. The church members did not call the teen fathers "unwed" fathers, "morally unworthy," or "welfare fathers." The teen fathers were not judged in the same way as the teen mothers. Nor did the counselors ask why it was the morally bad teen mothers who attended these meetings to improve their educational and social skills, not the teen fathers. The counselors themselves uttered not a word about the young men's morals, or the fact that, given the ages of the teen mothers, the men had committed statutory rape.

Teen fathers were almost invisible at the Center. Seldom did teen fathers take part in any of these programs. In an effort to make more fathers interested in the program, the Center changed the program's name from "Teen Mothers" to "Teen Parents." The Center's staff also developed a program, led by three men counselors, specifically geared to Black teen fathers. Occasionally one or two would visit the Center and sit in on a meeting or two, but not on any consistent basis or in any numbers. The counselors finally terminated the program within a month because so few men attended the meetings.

One major problem for these teenage mothers, which the counselors unwittingly supported and were unable to change (even with all of their expertise), was the weight of the morally deviant stigma. It was this stigma that hindered the counselors' ability to respond more positively to the teen mothers. It may have been easier for the counselors to retain a predominantly moral deviant view of the teen mothers, rather than become allies with the teen mothers. This position made sense to the counselors because, as they reminded me so often, their livelihood depended on agency funding and community support. To be fair, these counselors had no way of understanding the complexity of the teen mothers' experiences and had learned no way to respond to the concerned White mothers or to the school teachers in support of these mothers other than to teach the teen mothers to be quiet (as girls are silenced in school).

Chapter Nine

Creating the Potential for Growth

If I was a normal person, I wouldn't have to go through this. There just ain't no one to help me.

Sixteen-year-old De Vonya Smalls

According to a now-familiar African proverb, It takes a whole village to grow a child. A child thrives through connection and community. Yet the teen mothers I saw on a daily basis for more than three years did not have the support of such a village community. Instead, their early childhood "poverty of relationship" led to problems during adolescence. They had little or no support from the school, parents, extended family, social service agencies, or society at large before, during, or after their pregnancies. Even before De Vonya Smalls became pregnant, serious problems at home alienated her so much from her family that she sought comfort in the arms of another teenager. De Vonya wanted and needed a whole village to help her grow.

In this ethnographic study of De Vonya Smalls and others like her, I have sought to understand the past and current challenges facing these young mothers. My claim that gender, race, and class are integral to their experience has been borne out by evidence of the complex issues at play in their compromised lives. By moving beyond theories about the "culture of poverty," economic determinism, and "Black cultural strategies," I have been able to show how gender, race, and class interact to affect Black teenage mothers confronted by the structural forces and relational impoverishment in their immediate surroundings.

Rethinking the Explanations of Black Teenage Pregnancy

How do Moynihan's culture-of-poverty, Wilson's economic determinist, and Stack's cultural strategies theory fail to deepen our understanding of these teenage mothers' experiences?[1] Moynihan assumes that Black families are pathologically entangled in a culture of poverty. He maintains that the female-headed household reproduces a poverty culture because mothers are responsible for forming their children's values, whereas two-parent households with male breadwinners reproduce values favored by the middle class because they provide a different socialization, one that equips children with sufficient skills. But if underclass culture is such an overriding determinant in the social reproduction of Black teenage motherhood, what accounts for the similarity in the experiences of De Vonya Smalls and Diane Harris or of Lois Patterson and Evie Jenkins? De Vonya and Evie were from very different social classes and family backgrounds and had disparate educational and occupational opportunities during two distinct decades in the Black community's economic history. Yet both ended up in the same place and in much the same way, an outcome Moynihan's theory cannot explain.

Wilson's theory of economic determinism can differentiate some, but not all, of De Vonya's and Evie's experiences. Oakland and Richmond were far more vital and productive when seventeen-year-old Evie became pregnant in 1962 than when fifteen-year-old De Vonya became pregnant in 1985. As Wilson suggests, our nation's economic upheaval of the 1980s accounts for the high rates of unemployment among Black men and teenagers, widespread decreases in government funding for schools and housing (starting with the Reagan administration), escalating numbers of Black families headed by poor, or poorly paid, working women, increasing numbers of Black women on AFDC, decreasing numbers of Black extended family support systems, and increasing numbers of Black children who are poor. Wilson argues that reestablishing the man's major role as provider would build up the two-parent family and thus solve the problems caused by economic upheaval. He is partly right. But by not taking gender and structure into account and by not making women central to his thesis, Wilson upholds a patriarchal and class interpretation of lower-class Black teenage mothers. He does not adequately address the current structure of employment for Black women, like those in this study, which does not allow them to work at all, let alone pay them enough to provide for their families. Life is better if Black women can find jobs in which they earn enough not to have to depend on welfare or men wage earners. But more important, women's lives would be improved if motherhood were not assumed to be a woman's crowning achievement and if families headed by women were accorded the same power and prestige as families headed by men.

This limitation of Wilson's theory allows us to remain ignorant of other factors as well. Both sexist ideologies and inadequate support systems obstruct teen mothers' desires to acquire education and realize the American Dream—thus reproducing a generation of poor, dependent women. This limitation in his thinking is revealed as he quotes another social scientist to support his argument: "In the ghetto, the meaning of the illegitimate child is not ultimate disgrace. There is not the demand for abortion or for surrender of the child that one finds in more privileged communities. In the middle class, the disgrace of illegitimacy is tied to personal and family aspirations. In lower-class families, on the other hand, the girl loses only some of her already limited options by having an illegitimate child. On the contrary, a child is a symbol of the fact that she is a woman, and she may gain from having something of her own."[2]

Wilson's study does not take into account the fact that when teenage girls become mothers they experience deep depressions and other health problems, besides losing out on the already minuscule educational and job opportunities accorded Black women. Nor does Wilson's study account for the feelings people have about themselves and others when they have to make do with little, help others with even less, or depend on those with few resources themselves. Relationships occurring under such circumstances have small chance of being rich or productive, as relationships do when more resources are at the person's disposal. Wilson's study does not comprehend how painful it was to Susan Carter or Shana Leeds to watch alliances with their parents, friends, counselors, and teachers unravel when they became pregnant. Nor does Wilson realize the extent to which teenage mothers can feel disgraced by teenage motherhood or its effects on their personal aspirations and the aspirations of their mothers.

Standing between Moynihan's culture-of-poverty theory and Wilson's economic determinist model is Stack's assumption that certain cultural norms can overcome the hardship of poverty. Using an ethnographic method, Stack explores how people manage despite their economic hardship. However, her cultural approach is limited to a race and class framework. According to Stack, Black families make up for their economic hardship with "survival strategies" that involve family members and others. Like Wilson, Stack sees the problem as centered in the lack of jobs for men, although she (like Wilson) does concede that Black women need to work as well. Stack's work accomplishes two important tasks: she gives a good accounting of the strategies families used previously to survive tough times, and she vividly portrays the potency of the extended family in the 1970s and the contributions various members made to each other.

De Vonya and the other teen mothers in this study demonstrate quite clearly that the extended family no longer exists in its earlier form or with its former potency. Only one teen, Terry Parks, had an extended family she could consider supportive, but that support was woman-based, and she wanted support from a male. Lois Patterson's extended family was more a hindrance than a support. In the teen mothers' experience, extended families were both supportive and obstructive: what they gave with one hand, they took away with the other.

The theoretical formulations of Wilson and the cultural strategies of Stack, insightful and thought-provoking as they are, do not fully account for the ways women and teen mothers contribute to and are forced to create strategies against the ideologies and structures that oppress them. These Black adolescent girls in this study have been abandoned by the educational system and locked out of the job market. They offer a more complex view of Black families than most sociological assessments, in which Black families often appear as either deviant or saintly, but seldom as real as these girls portrayed them. They not only experience this complicated reality but also understand they can vividly describe how they experience these structural ucts and constraints. At the same time, they are deprived of other critical knowledge. Like the adolescent girls in Carol Gilligan's study, these girls are deprived of information about their bodies and sexuality that is critical to their decision making.

The interviews in this study eloquently demonstrate that these young women are not exhibiting lower-class or pathological behavior, as Moynihan and others believe. Rather, the lives of poor and middle-class Black teenage mothers add complexity to the structural perspective, providing rich evidence that they are not the "other," as the culture-of-poverty literature suggests. Each of these theories offers a limited perspective.

If we look to feminist theory again, we can see its contribution and its shortcomings regarding Black teenage mothers. In the past two decades feminist theory has moved the analysis of gender beyond the experiences of White women by bringing Black women's experiences from the margin to the center. But these insights have not been extended to much of the research on Black teenage mothers. Notions that do not threaten the status quo's assessments of failed adolescents lie at the center of much research on Black teenage mothers, and such notions then shape further research and political agencies.

The teen mothers in this study have been abandoned by an educational system that cannot offer them a safe environment conducive to learning, let alone the instruments of learning they need. Their teachers do not have the administrative, community, and financial support necessary to provide uncrowded classrooms in which respect for the other is fostered and excitement about learning is possible. The students do not have up-to-date textbooks, paper supplies, or equipment and training for our computer age. In addition, the schools do not provide girls with an educational environment in which they are perceived to be other than sexual objects.

The Poverty of Relationships: Linking Gender, Race, and Class

In attempting to comprehend the struggles of these teenagers as they face the usual adolescent tasks combined with pregnancy, we must ask, How do their relationships become impoverished through the interlinking of gender, race, and class effects? Because gender and race were constant in this study, class was the principal variable affecting the way these teenage mothers viewed their situation. When their description of their lives is held up to the light, it becomes clear that gender as well as race and class acted as a structured and psychological restraint on the teenage mothers' ability to move forward before, during, and after their pregnancies. The possibilities open to these teenage girls were limited structurally beginning in early childhood.

The Effects of Gender Inequality

Mainstream rhetoric expounds that girls as well as boys should be educated to succeed in life. The reality is quite different. At an early age, these teen mothers are forsaken by the schools in a variety of ways. They do not have physically safe classrooms in which respect for girls is fostered. They are perceived as and expected to behave as purely sex objects, or they are forgotten and left unprotected because teachers (and men in power) do not believe young Black girls need to concern themselves with acquiring a good education and securing long-term careers; after all, their main concern in life is really having babies and collecting welfare checks.

Sixteen-year-old De Vonya was living in a community that was sinking under the weight of drugs and gang violence at the same time as she was facing the challenges of one of the most significant stages in her life—adolescence and her burgeoning sexuality. No one gave De Vonya information about her body or sexuality; her mother believed that De Vonya would have construed the giving of such information as permission, even encouragement, to engage in sexual relations. Withholding information about sex ensured that De Vonya would remain a "nice girl," the kind of girl who would follow "moral" rules not to engage in sexual activity before marriage. But she was also learning from her peers and the media that being sexy and having sex was "cool."

At the same time, De Vonya began to lack relationships essential to her physical and mental development. She was unable to have a meaningful relationship based on trust and love with her father or, later, with her mother. Nor did she receive any support from the counselors or her baby's father. As a result, she did not learn what she should receive from others in her life. Girls who do not learn that they have the right to receive from others become underachievers, not just academically but socially and emotionally as well. De Vonya was doomed to teenage motherhood not because she was morally unrestrained but because she was unable to articulate who she was or what she needed and wanted out of life until she became focused on being a mother. She did not know how relationships with others could work for mutual good.

De Vonya serves to illustrate the interrelationship of two cultural trends. First, current research shows that the decline of adolescent girls' academic achievement that we have seen in recent decades is correlated with other profound changes in adolescents' biological clocks and interpersonal environments. These changes, such as the earlier occurrence of menarche (the beginning of sexual identity), combined with the lack of sex education and the overt and covert sexual harassment that often leads to early sexual relationships and abuse, make greater demands on girls today than in the 1950s and 1960s. Second, we have restricted children's and adolescents' knowledge of the maturation process and their sexuality. That children and adolescents, especially girls, are kept ignorant about the developmental process does not foster competence and maturity; rather, it fosters complacency and helplessness. It also puts our adolescent girls at risk, for without knowledge and critical thinking skills, our girls cannot learn to make responsible choices that will ultimately keep them safe.

To make matters more complicated, as De Vonya (like other girls) was beginning to develop physically, she was facing a perplexing double standard: with her development came sanctions against sexual freedom, while young men who were also experiencing adolescent development were granted the right to sexual freedom, from which they inferred the right to access teen girls' bodies. The admonishment to be a "nice girl" collided with the strategies of young men who counted on nice girls to "cave in" to such strategies: real men have sex no matter how they get it. Along with these problems, De Vonya, like other Black teenage girls, began to see little chance of acquiring a decent education, stable employment, marriage, and a comfortable family home—the American Dream.

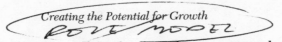

De Vonya did not have strong family and community relationships in which she could learn about intimacy and trust. Nor did she have someone to guide her through adolescence, helping her learn about herself as a girl and about her impending adulthood. That kind of guidance might have given her the foundation she needed to avoid the pitfalls of early motherhood.

De Vonya's mother had her own set of problems. Mary Smalls was barely staying on top of her own life, let alone her teenage daughter's life. Like other adult mothers she was confused about what and how much to tell her daughter about her sexuality, for she certainly did not want De Vonya to replicate her life. Yet because Mary Smalls's economic and emotional resources were depleted and she had so little control over her daughter's outcome, she could not stop De Vonya's life from moving in that direction.

The Effects of Race and Class

At the time when teenage pregnancies began to increase in the Black community, devastating workplace changes were occurring. Jobs were becoming scarce for many workers, public housing projects were beginning to appear in the community, pushing more people into less space, and mom and pop stores were moving out. Blacks were finding it more and more difficult to find and keep traditional jobs because of the sweeping economic changes occurring everywhere. Many laborers found themselves replaced by cheaper labor. White women began taking service jobs. Jobs ordinarily done by teenagers, such as paper deliveries, baby-sitting, and clerking at local stores, were taken over by adults. Finding themselves with no future, Black girls refocused their attention away from school and onto personal relationships.

Social reproduction theory assumes that those in power will reproduce the system that gave them power. This theory can be applied to the Black community inversely: those not in power will reproduce a powerless society. The exclusion of Black teenagers from the labor pool ensures that the social reproduction is effective, because it means that the Black community's labor pool will eventually shrivel up. The Black labor pool does not now, and may not in the future, consist of a skilled youthful population to replace its mothers and fathers as workers. This fact guarantees that the Black community will not be a productive economic and political force in the future. This examination of the labor market focuses primarily on how racism and class inequality have contributed to Black teenage motherhood. Gender also becomes a factor when we realize that girls can be shut out of the labor market quite easily because of the difference between rhetoric and reality.

Linking Gender, Race, and Class Inequalities

How do gender, race, and class play out in the lives of middle-class teenage mothers like Diane Harris and Evie Jenkins? Their interviews convinced me that we were looking at more than behavioral or structural problems of lower-class Black adolescent girls. Diane and Evie did not experience poverty, but they did not know much about their sexuality or about dealing with the men they met. Nor did they think that they had much of a future, because of the kind of jobs held by their mothers. It becomes clear from the interviews these Black girls lacked relationships essential to the physical and mental development they needed to accomplish during adolescence. Adolescence is a time when healthy and strong relationships with teachers, counselors, parents, and others in society are crucial.

It is during preadolescence and adolescence that girls learn about their sexuality. What the adolescent girls in this study learn from boys is merely that they are sexual. But they do not learn in a healthy way that menarche means the beginning of womanhood, and that it is a special time of celebration for them. Adequate discussion about their physical and emotional development is almost nonexistent, because the ideology in the larger society and the conservativism of the Black community prohibit frank discussions about sexuality.

The break between intimacy and trust noted by Carol Gilligan begins at an early age, when structural forces and patriarchal ideology coincide—men who cannot provide for their families can leave them without staining their own moral reputation.[3] To some degree, class influences these father-daughter relationships. The daughter of middle-class parents, Diane Harris had a strong relationship with her father. In telling about that relationship, Diane makes gender as well as class an issue. Poor and working-class teen mothers, such as De Vonya

Smalls, Terry Parks, and Shana Leeds, were unable to establish an intimate relationship with their fathers, although they wanted to do so.

These girls who were not able to establish relationships based on trust and intimacy with their fathers were not able to do so with other adults in their lives: their own mothers, their teachers, their counselors, or their babies' fathers.

The teenage girls in this study who lacked such pivotal relationships end up using denial to cover up deep relational problems that, if not solved, continue to burden the girls as they grow into womanhood. Mothers who, like Mary Smalls, were unable to resolve their own problems as teenagers did not learn how to help their daughters when they encountered similar problems during adolescence; nor did they see how these problems crossed the generations. Mary Smalls, at fifty-two, did not understand the process of sexual development herself. She grew up in a time and a culture in which women were not supposed to be concerned with their sexuality. That knowledge would be gained after they were safely married. Janet Carter, sixteen years younger than Mary and a nurse's aide with some understanding of sexuality, was also unsure of how to handle those issues with her daughter. Once again, it seems, as Carol Gilligan suggests in her work on middle-class girls, that in a patriarchal structure a woman's purity is part of her capital, as Diane Harris understood. A woman who wants a successful marriage stays a virgin or hides her sexual activity by not having children. The teen mothers did not have relationships with women who might help them sort out the process of adolescence and to understand new strategies for living a more productive teenage experience. Teachers and counselors backed off from handing these girls information regarding their sexuality. They preferred to stick to the status quo and to see these girls in class terms—as immoral lower-class girls. They upheld the views of social conservatives and some liberals whose agenda is to reassert the patriarchal family structure.

The patriarchical family structure was certainly important to the teen mothers. Diane cringed at the thought of losing her middle-class status and feared becoming like those "lower-class ghetto mentality girls." She longed for her childhood lifestyle and created through appearance what she currently missed. She wanted very much to repeat her "wonderful" relationship with her father, who died when she was young. Her unemotional mother could provide Diane only material comfort, not the emotional relationship she needed—she could not replace Diane's lost father. Diane's desire to repeat the life she had with her father was so compelling that she considered giving her son to his father because she believed that the kind of middle-class professional man she desired, who would give her back the middle-class status that set her apart from other Black teenage mothers, would not marry a teenage mother. Diane thus provides an example of the need to focus on class and gender as well as race in the analysis of teenage mothers' lives.

The interviews of older teen mothers such as Evie Jenkins are certainly crucial to understanding the interaction of gender, race, and class. Evie brings to the study a long-term memory of what it was for her to be a teenage mother twenty-five years before. We learn through her that relationships are important after the pregnancy, just as Diane tells us they are important before the pregnancy. We also learn that many Black families were not supportive of teenage pregnancy decades ago, just as Diane's story tells us that that attitude has not changed. Like Diane, Evie also paid a great price for being a teenage mother, having to become a welfare mother and thereby losing her middle-class status. She could not develop a maturing and healthy relationship with her mother at a critical time when, as Carol Gilligan believes, connection with others (especially women) is essential for the development of adolescent girls.

Evie's interview shows that her relationship with her mother was weakened by her pregnancy. She never recovered from the breakdown of that relationship. Nor did she establish any relationship at all with her father. Evie's story is therefore central to my thesis about the tremendous impact of teenage motherhood, especially in dismissing the idea that Black adult mothers condone teenage pregnancy. Her interviews allow us to build a bridge between the past and the future. If we had asked serious questions twenty-five years ago about teenage pregnancy and the connection between economic changes in the Black community and Black girls' adolescent development, perhaps we would not have this problem today.

The Motherhood Strategy

Why, then, did these teenage mothers have babies? If we use the village as a metaphor, we must say that in absence of support from the

members of a village, in which everyone pools their emotional and
economic resources, these teen mothers had babies because they
were isolated from society and unwanted by everyone around them.
In order for them to grow, they needed to be loved and nourished.
Without both, they created love where they could. These interviews
confirm De Vonya's revelation that motherhood is a strategy: "I can
be a mother if I can't be anything else."

In using the motherhood strategy, the teen mothers in this study
were not behaving pathologically, but were using the only survival
strategy they believed was available to them. With this strategy comes
the illusion of well-being. Indeed, these young women were trying to
impose order on their lives, a necessity completely unfamiliar to men
such as Moynihan. Tragically, in most cases, when teen mothers use
motherhood as a coping strategy and a means of feeling good about
themselves, they re-create the very circumstances they are seeking to
avoid.

In an urban environment dominated by drugs, gangs, delinquency,
and unemployment and having few supportive men, the teenage girls
in this study used motherhood to establish an alternative lifestyle because they did not have the resources to enable them to grow up safely
and happily. When Shana Leeds said, "He loved me and left," she described both her father and her baby's father.

All of the teen mothers thought motherhood would bring them love
and happiness. Some believed motherhood gave them middle-class
stability. Others thought it gave them a focus in their lives, providing
them with a sense of belonging and, perhaps, the means to find what
they so urgently needed—security and protection. De Vonya Smalls
wanted motherhood to make up for her own mother's lack of love for
her. Susan Carter used motherhood in her struggle against the effects
of childhood sexual abuse. Terry Parks compensated for being over involved with female love and for the loss of her father by identifying
with the Brady Bunch, a patriarchal television family, and by thinking
that her son would give her "male love." Diane Harris, Evie Jenkins,
Lois Patterson, and Shana Leeds wanted motherhood to turn them
into "something special" in the eyes of the babies' fathers.

The motherhood strategy shows that these mothers had some sense
of dignity as they yearned to have control over their lives. These young

women were aware of the standards and actions required of them by their families and friends. Except for those who admitted they had babies to make up for what they perceived to be their own maternal deprivation, most of these teen mothers felt that they were not doing anything other than just being teenagers and mothers and students, struggling to succeed.

In contrast to the goals of this motherhood strategy, when these Black teenage girls became mothers they were surprised by the general reaction to their pregnancy and found themselves ambushed by a welfare system, stigmatized, and forced to cheat and lie in order to bring stability and order into their lives.

Strategies of Resistance:
Reconstructing Relationships

What the teen mothers said about their lives made me appreciate David Morgan's notion of the "dance of agency and structure."[4] This concept assumes that people actively create strategies to deal with structural forces that may be in their way and explains how people without much power deal with a powerful system. The teen mothers did so by suggesting that while they could not fend off the structural forces at play in their lives, they used their wits to try to escape from their situation. De Vonya insisted, "I ain't goin' let happen to me what happened to my mother." De Vonya was determined to get an education and fulfill her dreams while being a teen mother.

In a variety of ways sixteen-year-old De Vonya rejected the stereotype that she was sexually permissive. She pointed to the steady relationship she initially had with Matthew, her need for commitment from him and her father, and her commitment to mainstream values—college education and monogamous relationships. But De Vonya and the teen mothers also offset the stereotypes about them by using the same labels against other teen mothers. They were quite capable of espousing similar views about other teen mothers' moral values and categorizing them as "good," "not so bad," and "really bad" girls—distinguishing the "it was an accident" type from the "ghetto mentality" type. Like most of us, the teen mothers judged girls who were not teen welfare mothers as "good," short-term teen welfare mothers as "not so bad," and long-term teen welfare mothers as "really bad." That teen mothers should do the same moral pegging as those who peg them is not surprising. Most people live in accordance with mainstream norms and moral values in order to belong to a community of people. If we do not obtain a sense of self-worth through the community, we tend to build one up for ourselves.

De Vonya, who was the daughter of a former teenage mother, may have been repeating her mother's experiences by becoming an impoverished teenage mother herself. But her mother, calling on her own experiences, tried as best she could to stop her daughter from following in her footsteps, by warning her daughter not to have sex until she married, checking on her daughter's menstrual cycles, and using her life as a negative example. That Mary Smalls and other adult mothers failed to dissuade their daughters from becoming young mothers raises questions about what strategies might work.

Another strategy to prevent unwed motherhood was the grandmothers' acknowledgment that their sons had fathered the babies. These grandmothers show how intervention is possible and suggest that the gathering of women in support of other women may help, even if they do not bring about the long-term involvement of the fathers with their babies. Another strategy that worked to some degree was Terry and Dana's housing arrangement. Terry felt this living arrangement was imperfect since it could be disrupted at any time. Also, she did not value it as much as she would have valued a man-centered family.

Intervention in the generational cycle of early mothering and poverty was also attempted by people of the community who tried to develop professional programs to help these mothers learn parenting and job skills. The peer meetings gave the teen mothers a chance to see others in similar situations and to talk about and understand their lives. But the counselors undermined these lessons with their own deeply rooted traditional gender and class values. As a result, neither the counselors nor the teen mothers attempted to address problems related to gender and class. When teen mothers became pregnant a second time, the counselors withdrew from them, depriving them of the counselors' assistance and contact with other teen mothers with similar problems, instead of trying to understand what factors might have led to the second pregnancy.

This study demonstrates how people respond to institutional oppression by developing their own strategies. Some strategies worked, and others did not.

The Consequences

What did the teen mothers think about being teen mothers? More than three-quarters of the thirty-two teen mothers said they regretted having a baby at such a young age. De Vonya Smalls's response was typical: "I wish I hadn't gotten pregnant when I did. But I want to finish school and go to college. So when it's time to marry, I still has the ability to get a job. I won't have to depend on nobody, not even my husband, for money."

"If you had to live your life over again, what would you change?" I asked De Vonya.

"I would not get pregnant," she said with a nervous laugh. "That's what I would change."

She sighed. She may have been disappointed with motherhood because, as one counselor noted, "The teen mothers expect that their babies will love them immediately." But babies need far more love from their mothers than they can give. Teen mothers experience bitter disappointment when they do not receive the love they expect from their babies. Motherhood puts tremendous demands upon the mothers' time, energy, and emotions, demands for which they are not prepared. In response they may withdraw or become angry or depressed. This lays the ground for emotional maternal deprivation for the infants, setting the stage for later developmental problems. Although the teen mothers in this study made great efforts to be "good" mothers, Terry Parks admitted during one of my visits that she "loves little babies but not when they grow up, past two." This point is not a condemnation of the teen mothers. Rather, I suggest that at this age and stage of adolescent development, a time when adolescent girls need tremendous support to handle the physical and emotional changes they inevitably experience, a teen mother may not be able to push aside her own needs to be mothered in order to adequately mother her own child.

I suspect the daughters' needs for further mothering—to become daughters again—cannot be satisfied by their adult mothers.[5] The adult mothers in this study could not afford to keep mothering their teenage daughters, economically, socially, or emotionally. De Vonya answered my question, "What advice do you have for teenagers who are thinking about becoming mothers?" by leaning over me to yell into the microphone: "Don't have no babies! They should think about it before they do because it's a lot of responsibility and changes your life a lot. It cost a lot of money and you can't get up and go no more like when your friends come and you want to go somewhere to the movies. Gotta think about if the father's going to stay around and a lot of different things." Judging by the number of Black teenage girls who become pregnant each year, De Vonya's warnings might fall on deaf ears. It is possible that teenage girls can hear all about the problems of teenage motherhood and yet still be lured by the promise of motherhood's supposed omnipotence.

The Teen Mothers' Last Words

The last time I visited De Vonya, she was carrying La Shetta in one arm while wheeling the stroller with the other, moving toward the bus stop for a trip to the welfare office. I asked her what she thought would help other teenage girls avoid some of the problems she had encountered: "You need someone who really knows. . . . If I would have had someone to talk to, someone who really knows how it is . . . But there was really no one like that I knew. When you talked about support groups and stuff like that, now I want them even more. It's just good to have someone to finally talk to about it. If I was a normal person, I wouldn't have to go through this. There just ain't no one to help me."

"There just ain't no one to help me." When I called her again, De Vonya's telephone had been disconnected. The "penthouse" seemed empty when I stopped by there.

Shortly after I concluded these interviews, I called each young mother, trying to visit each of them one last time. Evie Jenkins was still feeling "poorly" and looked tired when I saw her last. Diane Harris and her family had moved to Seattle, according to the person living in her old apartment. Lois Patterson was in the process of moving when I visited her, and we wrapped her children's jelly jars in newspapers as we talked about her new apartment in yet another depleted neighborhood. Susan Carter and Shana Leeds had simply disappeared. One might say that Terry Parks and Dana Little were doing better than most of the others, with the exception of Diane Harris. Terry and Dana were comfortably settled into their apartment, although they still had to hope that their living arrangement would not come to the attention of their social worker. Terry said with a quiver in her voice, "Why should they care? We're doing what we can."

Implications for the Future:
Strategies for Change

While this study is small and limited to a particular region of the country, its findings refute the popular view, as expressed, for example, by the journalist Mary McGrory: "Illegitimacy has pretty much lost its sting in certain ghetto neighborhoods, therefore, we need to stigmatize it again."[6] The teen mothers suggest that teenage motherhood does, in fact, "sting," as it stigmatizes both the teenage mother and her mother. This research shows that we need to develop a more sophisticated understanding of the adolescent process for Black girls, and it shows the way gender relations and socioeconomic conditions affect these teenage girls' lives and the way society's beliefs about moral values influence their relationships.

The young Black women in this study are like most Black women today. They want the traditional American Dream—education, a family, and a home. They do not reject the idea of marrying before having a baby, as many of today's White women do. I thought about the facetiousness of the morally superior "good girl" when a White teenager told me that she became sexually active at thirteen. She liked boys, she said, but she did not plan on being with anyone at this time of her life. As she put it, "I learned everything I could about me and birth control because I didn't want to become pregnant by him."

The erroneous belief that nice girls do not engage in sex demonstrates the power of the male culture of protection I mentioned earlier. The men who have sexual relations with these "bad" girls escape the sanction experienced by the teen mothers because, according to the double standard, girls are blamed for promiscuity, not boys. The irony here is that while White women might flaunt their autonomy and the independence of traditional values and are accepted and even admired by some people for doing so, Black women who do not act according to traditional values, even though they desire to, are blamed. The teen mothers in this study were anxious to fight that stereotype; they wanted me to see them as "regular old ladies," to strongly reject the popular stereotype of them as "welfare cheats," and to counter the image that they were immoral and irresponsible.

The issue of moral values is an extremely important one for these teen mothers, as well as for all Black mothers, since the image of deviant mothers raising deviant children incites politicians to call for the end of welfare and other social policies. In the current political climate, welfare opponents argue that taxpayers should not support social policies for so-called immoral Black teenage mothers. This study proposes that just family policies to assist teenage mothers and their adult mothers are vital to these mothers, as evidenced by the problems the teen mothers reported and by my findings that socioeconomic strains aggravate these problems.

The other side of the American Dream, which we fail to emphasize as often as we should, is the belief that our communities should rise to the aid of all its members. In that American Dream, people think not only of themselves and their families but also of their connection to others in their community. In communities with that focus, adolescents do not need to create fantasies of the good life based on television families. Nor do they have to use motherhood as a way to gain love and support.

Liberals and feminists who are concerned about teenage girls have the opportunity to offer support to these girls. So far, they have failed to comprehend the experiences of Black teenage mothers and to act upon them with the same vigor they give to White women's issues and to Black men's employment issues. Not all liberals and feminists ignore teenage mothers. Liberals have made some attempt to understand the issues these young girls face, and they have been determined in their efforts to find workable strategies, but so far they have failed to grasp the complexity of these issues.[7] The same can be said for many but not all feminists. While feminists familiar with the plight of Black teenage mothers support studies such as this, many are not comfortable addressing these issues. Although they may not want to admit it, they ignore the fact that Black girls, like all women, suffer the consequences of certain stereotypical images: to cite only three, they are passive, they can be treated as sexual objects, and they are responsible primarily for raising children. By ignoring how gender, race, and class play out in the lives of Black adolescent girls and adolescent mothers, feminists have failed to put into practice what they write regarding equality for all women. The few feminists who speak up do so privately. Most tell me that they want to extend their research and political agenda further, but they cannot, they say in whispered voices, because they are afraid of being called racist if they dare suggest a new way to see Black women.

There is no question that activists, both feminists and those interested in the Black community, do tremendously important work concerning how women's poverty and lack of employment opportunities contribute to the problems of women in the Black community. But they often make these observations without adequately exploring how deeply these problems affect Black teenage girls. Black teenage girls' experiences are rarely understood as part of the larger economic and social shifts in the lives of teenagers, women, and Americans in general. Consequently, the analysis of Black women's situations stops at an analysis of racism. When Black teenage mothers are written off as morally deviant, liberals and feminists can call for an end to racism, discuss the loss of extended families, the problems of being poor in America, and the need to end sexist attitudes, and yet neglect to explore the same influences in the experiences of Black teenage mothers. That so many feminists ignore the plight of Black adolescent girls suggests they do not see teenage motherhood as having anything to do with gender inequality. If we continue to ignore the experiences of Black adolescent girls, the Black community stands a very good chance of declining even further.

A Good Enough Village in Which to Grow

The teen mothers' perceptions of their adolescent years make eight issues very clear. First, these teen mothers' experiences show that teen girls need guidance in the early years of preadolescence and adolescence, especially before the age of fifteen. As early as age five, girls should begin learning as much about their bodies as they are able to comprehend. The level of girls' knowledge about their emotional and physical development could be enhanced each year so that by the end of preadolescence girls have sufficient knowledge about their sexuality.

Second, more research is needed concerning girls' preadolescence so that we can increase our awareness of that experience and see if there are possibilities for changing girls' negative pubescent experiences. For example, how might the literature incorporate what girls think about the changes in themselves and the challenges in their social lives? How can their parents contribute to this stage of their daughters' development? How can the teen mothers' experiences expand our theoretical understanding of girls' internal and external worlds during these vulnerable years? Further study of girls' preadolescent shifts and demands can tell us what effective support systems might aid girls as they make the transition from preadolescence to adolescence to adulthood.

Third, the strategies used by the teen mothers of this study to achieve some kind of support system show that a support system is essential as teens go through adolescence. Even if family support is not available, alternative support groups would benefit the girls' social and emotional development, even during preadolescence. One such benefit might be to develop the confidence of girls during this earlier period. I would like to see organizations such as the Girl Scouts, Girls Inc., the YWCA, and other community-based centers offer support groups for girls and places to meet regularly. Since it takes money to bring about any kind of change, these groups could use some of the donations they raise to launch neighborhood-based girls' groups. The members of these community groups could act as role models and mentors for these girls. In this setting girls would be able to talk about their disappointments and challenges, their relationships with boys, and sexual abuse, as well as the joys and happiness they experience. They would be able to learn social skills for handling loss and for establishing trust with appropriate persons.

Libraries could offer reading groups led by informed adults or older teen volunteers where girls could discuss issues raised in teenage romance novels, movies about teenage girls, or teenage magazines, thus learning about themselves and how to interact with others, including boys. Organizations such as Planned Parenthood could provide teenage girls meeting space as well as guest speakers to discuss sexual issues.

The support systems promoted by the Black and feminist communities could ensure that educational and political support for adolescent girls is also available. In doing so, they could influence the educational systems to rethink their teaching strategies for Black girls and require for all students classes on sexuality geared toward understanding preadolescence and adolescence. These schools could provide space for girls to meet in peer groups and interact with older teenagers who might share their knowledge of the Black teenage culture and communication while also helping the younger teens learn to see the world from a larger perspective. Young teens could also benefit from learning what constitutes healthy relationships with boys and how to develop them. (They could also provide space for mothers of teenage girls who may need to talk and learn about adolescence.)

Fourth, just as girls need to rethink their notions about femininity and motherhood, boys need to change their distorted notions about masculinity and fatherhood. A greater effort could be made to help boys understand how their ideas and behavior are detrimental to themselves as well as to young women. (Rap songs, with lyrics such as "Women ain't nothin but bitches to be screwed" by Black rap artists 2 Live Crew, demonstrate the depth of the problem for Black adolescent girls.) Through such a new understanding they could acquire a healthy sense of manhood. Educational classes, job training programs, and a focus on the benefits of interacting with women in a positive way rather than as sexual objects would provide needed support to both young men and young women.

Fifth, the welfare system could do more than give out small sums of money to poor mothers. A number of policies regarding family support systems could be enacted. For instance, eligibility workers could be retrained to see themselves as supporters, to be empathetic, to offer real job training, and to seek more economic and emotional support for the entire family unit. They could start by changing their attitudes and their pejorative treatment of girls and by incorporating the whole family, including the grandmothers, grandfathers, and the babies' fathers, into social policies.

Sixth, those involved in this new social support system can let teen mothers help decide how much support is needed, and they can develop the needed resources in concert. The teen mothers in this study want a community consisting of fully present and fully responsible adults to protect them and help them prepare for successfully living in the world.

Seventh, Blacks and feminists can do a great deal for these Black teenage mothers by putting them on their agendas when they conduct research and work to enact programs for families, work, gender and race equality, and economic parity. They can stress to politicians the need for money and information in creating programs for adolescent girls. Feminists, liberals, and conservatives would do well to realize that the moral evaluation of teenage mothers as deviant is inaccurate and that such disparagement does nothing but exacerbate already intractable problems.

We can learn a great deal from the telephone caller quoted at the beginning of this ethology, who blamed Black adolescent girls for the social problems of the entire Black community. His statements exemplify the hypocrisy of our American society. We profess to love and care for all children and promote the kind of family values that emphasize being supportive of children. But we often treat poor children and adolescents, especially Black adolescents, as if all of them are delinquents and unworthy of the same kind of love and care we give to White middle-class preadolescent boys.

Rather than take Black girls under our wings as they grow, we consider them grown up when they become adolescents, or, worse, we consider them adversaries. Too often we cease to love and care; instead, we seek to control these adolescent girls, not to provide them the knowledge and skills they need to function successfully in the adult world toward which they are moving. We have the idea that we must separate from our children as they grow up. We have not learned to live in a society of mutuality and interdependence. In our ever more needful world, we may not always be able to be our sisters' (or brothers') keepers, but we can bring about the social change and the guidance necessary to support Black teenage girls' strategies for impending adulthood that are far better than engaging in premature sex and becoming mothers at age fifteen.

The eighth strategy, and, I suggest, the most important one for feminists, will be to demonstrate to young Black girls the compromising ramifications of upholding a masculinist, patriarchal, and ethnocentric model of family life in which men are expected to have all the jobs, money, and power. Feminists can show these girls that in that kind of family life little girls will not learn power-enhancing strategies to lead independent lives. Without those strategies, little girls learn to need male love, to let men dictate the timing of sexual relations, to hide sexual abuse, and to let men walk away without taking responsibility for their actions. Feminists can be instructive as well in showing how the women-headed family life their mothers have organized merits respect and support from the wider society.

As suggested by those teenage mothers who regret having their babies, negative views about Black teenage mothers also threaten the positive development of their children. Such babies need their mothers and others to value them within our American village. Since politicians are not swayed by sentiment and are usually not swayed by the circumstances of Black teenage mothers, we may expect that without increased financial resources, family policies, and support from social service agencies to rebuild extended families (as Terry and Dana attempted to do), these mothers will continue to experience alienation and failure. The tragic consequence of such a social scenario will be the further erosion of the support system of Black teenage mothers' families and the Black community in general.

As this study demonstrates, we can develop such a village for Black teenage mothers, their children, and their families, a complex and beneficial framework of "good enough" support, if a gender, race, and class perspective is used to explore the meaning of their experiences. After all, these teenage mothers are moving inexorably toward adulthood and are raising the children who are the future's Black adults. The future of the Black community depends, as does American society, on respect for differences and on equality of opportunity not just to survive but to thrive. It is not just these Black teenage mothers, but each of us, who needs a village in which to grow.

Appendixes

Appendix A
Background of the Study

In this study I have let the material direct the interpretation; it gave me a sense of "What's going on out there." That is, I used induction—drawing conclusions and hypotheses from the data. My methodology has been influenced by the work of Anselm Strauss, Ann Oakley, and Shulumit Reinharz.[1] Anselm Strauss's discussion of the value of qualitative analysis and delineation of the complexities involved in an issue, particularly the traditional emphasis of the Chicago school of sociology on the need for "grasping the actors' viewpoints for understanding interaction, process, and social change,"[2] has strengthened my understanding of the issues.

Both Oakley's and Reinharz's use of feminist methodology has been the basis for my interviewing technique. I found Oakley's methodology most helpful. Oakley writes, "Where both interviewer and interviewee share membership of the same minority group, the basis for equality may impress itself even more urgently on the interviewer's consciousness." She uses an example from her own work on motherhood to show how the approach works. Like Oakley, I followed the practice of answering all personal questions and questions about the research as fully as was required. I also answered any advice questions as best I could based on my own experiences. As Oakley suggests about her own interviews, I think that the way I responded to the interviewees' questions and the casual atmosphere I tried to create may have encouraged them to regard me as more than an "instrument of data-collection."[3]

Reinharz sums up this method best when she maintains that by listening to women and understanding women's participation in particular social systems, and establishing the "distribution of phenomena accessible only through sensitive interviewing," feminist interview researchers have unveiled ignored or misinterpreted past universes of experience.[4] To me, qualitative feminist methodology is a way to bridge the gap between the literature's discussion of teenage mothers' experiences and their actual lived experiences.

My own experiences as a teen mother more than twenty years ago bring me closer to this subject than other researchers. As sociologist Troy Duster notes, the closer one is to the group under study, the more one can see the diversity. The further away, the more one sees the uniformity.[5] Being a teenage mother myself allowed me to ask different questions than other researchers and to see the complexity of the issue. But my own experiences served only as a jumping-off place. They led me to the ballpark. Once there, I had to rethink many of my own assumptions and go beyond my personal experiences. Their poverty was greater and their relationships with their families were sadder than my own.

I collected data from multiple sources—a method referred to as *triangulation* in the qualitative methodology literature. As Norman Denzin, an advocate of this method, claims, the researcher can simultaneously combine document analysis, respondent and informant interviewing, direct participation and observation, and introspection.[6] For example, I asked the counselors, "What do the teen mothers talk about most of the time?" In one way or another, most said, "their mothers' attitude," or, "the baby's father." Those comments helped me see that the teen mothers had repeatedly voiced their concerns about relational issues, thereby verifying their discussions with me.

One of the teen counselors provided me with additional background information. She went through her files to answer a short questionnaire I drew up on teenage mothers' family support networks, providing me information on thirty-five teen mothers who attended a youth program for teenage mothers in Richmond. An Oakland high school teacher gave me data from an unpublished report on teenage mothers in her school who reported being sexually abused in their early childhood. These responses supported my suggestion that the issue of sexual abuse of girls deserves serious attention from counselors and others who work with the teen mothers.

I developed a questionnaire of 126 items that asked the teen mothers about their experiences before, during, and after their pregnancies. I asked questions about various common conceptions: the idea of passive and promiscuous teenagers, the notion that the role of provider is the only important one for men in the lives of these women, the notion of strong cultural support for them as teenage mothers, the concept of extended family support networks, and the idea that the women had babies to receive welfare aid.

I transcribed the material verbatim except for names and other identifying markers, which were changed during the transcription. The transcriptions were then photocopied and shared with my Berkeley women's group during our weekly Saturday morning meetings at a small cafe on Hearst Street. The group consisted of women with educational backgrounds similar to mine in sociology and psychology. We met over the course of two years to talk about this project.

Each woman would discuss her take on the material and how it fit or did not fit with feminist theory and theories about Black women. After those discussions I would return home to record their impressions and any patterns discerned by the group. But mostly I worked alone, coding each teen mother on background variables and patterns and reading and rereading my field-notes, supporting documents, and relevant literature. I chose quotes that best represented the typical responses, overall categories, and major themes. I used quotes from the small sample of seven and the larger sample of thirty-two to include a wide range of responses.

I began to see the patterns, and I devised categories based on the teen mothers' descriptions and my own observations. There were many surprises that made me rethink some of my own assumptions. For example, in response to the question, "Did you confide in anyone when you found out you were pregnant?" I had expected the teen mothers, especially those still living with their mothers, to mention their mothers, but few did. I put the teen mothers' responses together with my observations and my interviews with the adult mothers, counselors, and others in these communities. I was able to use that material to generate my ideas about the teen mothers' relationships with their mothers. My interviews and the adult teen mothers' and the teen mothers' assessments of their mothers allowed me to generate two major categories of adult mothers based on their perceptions of the effects of teenage motherhood on their lives.

I followed a similar procedure regarding the teen mothers' answers to questions about their relations to men. I asked all the teen mothers questions such as, "Is [the baby's father] involved in your child's life?" "Would you like him to be more involved with your child?" They did not simply respond yes or no to these questions. Most went into great detail about their relationships with the babies' fathers. The question, "Age of your father when he had his first child?" prompted another kind of response. Most teen mothers said, "I don't know." This response prompted more questions about their fathers, which eventually provided the material on the teen mothers' relationships with their fathers and their babies' fathers. I also created three categories of babies' fathers: category 1 consisted of unemployed fathers, category 2 consisted of employed fathers, and category 3 consisted of teen fathers who married the teen mothers (all of these marriages ended in divorce). Within each category the teen mothers' responses to questions about their babies' fathers were also coded to determine whether they gave money for the children and were involved in their lives.

Questions such as, "How would you describe the quality of your life since you've been on AFDC?" caused most of the teen mothers to launch into a long discourse about those experiences. Their comments helped me understand the psychological toll on them and the energy they expended in responding to those experiences. Visits with them at various community gatherings and observations of them in group meetings helped confirm my theoretical assumption that effective strategies for change must start before girls reach adolescence and must include education, money, and emotional support for the girls and their families.

In seeking answers to questions about Black teenage mothers, I ask, How we might come to see them as whole human beings, not in part, and not as stereotypes? The larger sociological questions for me are addressed in these inquiries: How do people make sense of their lives and their social environment? Do they give up or give in to the pressures of living in adverse conditions? In what way do people alter these structural forces? How do they affect their environment, and under what conditions do they succeed or fail?

This book is not only about Black teenage mothers. It is also about a community—one that is under constant attack and surveillance for supposedly having substandard cultural and moral values—and how it deals with members who may reinforce the community's deviant image.

Appendix B
Questionnaire

SECTION 1. DEMOGRAPHICS

1. Name
2. Age
3. Residence
4. Religion
5. Education
6. Income
7. Source
8. Marital status
9. Children
10. Ages

SECTION 2. FAMILY INFORMATION

11. Mother's education
12. Father's education
13. Mother's religion
14. Mother's marital status
15. Father's marital status
16. Father's religion
17. Mother's annual income
18. Father's annual income
19. Number of siblings
20. Age of your mother when she had first child

21. Did your mother ever receive AFDC?
    a. If yes, how old were you when she applied?
    b. Did she stop receiving AFDC at any time?
    c. How old were you when she stopped?
    d. Why did she stop?
22. Did your mother work?
    a. If yes, how old were you when she went to work?
    b. What kind of work is she doing?
    c. Income from work?
    d. Did she stop working at any time?
       1. How old were you when she stopped?
       2. Why did she stop?
23. Did your mother receive income from other sources?
24. Age of your father when he had first child
25. Did your father work?
    a. If yes, how old were you when he worked?
    b. What kind of work did he do?
    c. Income from work?
    d. Did he stop working at any time?
       1. How old were you when he stopped working?
       2. Why did he stop working?
26. Did your father receive AFDC?
    a. If yes, how old were you when he applied for AFDC?
    b. How old were you when he stopped receiving AFDC?
    c. Why did he stop receiving AFDC?
27. Do you have sisters/brothers who receive AFDC?
28. Do you have sisters/brothers who are teenage parents?
29. If your parents received AFDC when you were growing up, what was that experience like for you?
30. If yes, what did they think about:
    a. Having to depend on AFDC?
    b. AFDC in general?
    c. About your experiences with AFDC?
31. If your parents did not receive AFDC when you were growing up, what did they think about:
    a. AFDC in general?
    b. Your experiences with AFDC?
    c. Other people who receive AFDC?
32. What did your (a) mother and (b) father say to you about:
    1. Getting off AFDC?
    2. Staying on AFDC?
    3. Family planning services?

33. What did your (a) mother and (b) father say to you about:
    1. Getting pregnant?
    2. Having the baby?
    3. Leaving or continuing in school?
    4. The baby's father?
34. What did your (a) mother and (b) father say to you about:
    1. Birth control?
    2. Abortion?
    3. Adoption?
    4. Getting married?
35. Did you confide in anyone when you found out you were pregnant?
    a. If so, who did you confide in?
    b. Who was the most supportive?
    c. Who was the least supportive?
    d. If not, why not?

SECTION 3. SEXUALITY

36. How old were you when you first thought about having children?
37. How old were you when you first thought about having sex?
38. How old were you when you first thought about using birth control?
39. How old were you when your parents first talked to you about sex?
40. What method of birth control are you using?

SECTION 4. MOTHERHOOD

41. How old were you when your child(ren) were born?
    a. First child
    b. Second
    c. Third
    d. Fourth
42. Did you want to have your child(ren)?
43. What is it like raising a child(ren) on welfare?
44. Do you think women have child(ren) in order to receive AFDC?
45. What do you think of teenagers who:
    a. Have sex?
    b. Have child(ren)?
    c. Are on welfare?
46. How many children do you want?
47. What do you receive from the child(ren)?
    a. Did you miss out on (the answer) when you were growing up?
    b. Why?

48. In what way do you think that your experiences as a mother are similar to or different from mothers who are not teenagers and on welfare?
49. Who are the male role models in your child(ren)'s lives?
50. What are your plans for your children?
    a. Schooling?
    b. Sex education?
    c. Other plans?
51. Will you have more children while you are on welfare?
    a. If yes, in what way do you think AFDC could be helpful?
    b. If no, why not?

SECTION 5. INFORMATION ON BABIES' FATHERS

52. Why didn't you marry the baby's father?
53. What is it like raising a child without a father?
54. How old was the child's father when his first child was born?
55. His educational level?
56. His religion?
    a. Does he attend church?
    b. If so, how often?
57. His occupation?
58. His income from work?
59. His income from other sources?
60. If no income, how does he support:
    a. Himself?
    b. Child(ren)?
    c. You?
61. Does he live (or has he ever lived) with you?
62. If no, is he involved in the child(ren)'s life?
    a. Does he visit?
    b. Is he emotionally supportive?
    c. Does he plan for the child(ren)'s future?
    d. Other?
63. If he is not involved at all, what would you think about the welfare agency locating him and making him take on some responsibility for the child(ren)?
    a. Would you want financial support?
    b. Would you want to resume the relationship?
64. What do you know about his family's background?
    a. Income?
    b. Education?

c. Occupation?
d. Religion?
e. Marital status?
f. Other relatives?

65. What kind of relationship does his family have with the child(ren)?
    a. Do they offer financial support? Specify.
    b. Do they offer emotional support? Specify.
66. What do they do and how often do they contribute to that support?
67. Are they (or have they ever) been on AFDC?
68. How do you feel about the child(ren)'s father?
69. Do you think he exerted pressure on you to have:
    a. Sex?
    b. Child(ren)?
70. If yes, exactly what did he do and why?
71. Why didn't he marry you?
72. What does he feel about:
    a. You?
    b. The child(ren)?
    c. Your lifestyle?
73. Did he offer you any emotional support?
    a. If yes, what did (or does) he do?
    b. If no, why not?
74. What does he think about:
    a. Birth control?
    b. Abortion?
    c. Adoption?
75. What did you expect from him as the father of your child?
    a. Did you call him or see him when you knew that you were pregnant?
    b. How did he react?
    c. Were you happy to share that experience with him?
    d. Did you blame him?
76. What do you think of the AFDC's program regarding fathers' child support?

SECTION 6. SCHOOL

77. What was school like for you?
78. What grade were you in when you became pregnant?
79. Did you have many friends?
80. What kind of grades did you receive?

81. Tell me about the relationship you had with the teachers.
82. Did you take sex education courses?
    a. If yes, what did you learn in the courses?
    b. If no, why not?
83. Are you attending school now?
    a. If yes, what kind of school?
    b. What kind of classes are you taking?
84. What do you think about being in school now?
85. If not attending school, why not?
86. What kind of child care arrangements do you have?
87. Who do you rely on for most support for child care?
88. How do you manage to attend school and raise a child at the same time?

SECTION 7. WELFARE

89. What was it like for you to apply for welfare?
90. How did you find out about the welfare program?
91. What was the process like:
    a. How did you apply?
    b. What kind of paperwork was required?
    c. What kind of waiting period?
92. Tell me about your relationship with your social worker.
93. How old were you when you formed your own household?
94. What kind of housing do you have at the present time?
    a. Do you have roommates?
    b. How many rooms do you have?
    c. How often have you moved, and why?
95. Tell me about the advantages of being on AFDC.
96. Tell me about the disadvantages of being on AFDC.
97. Have you ever been denied anything at all because you are:
    a. A teenage mother?
    b. A single parent?
    c. Young?
    d. Poor?
    e. On AFDC?
    f. Black?
    g. A woman?
98. Now, I would like to know how you budget your money. How much do you spend monthly on:
    a. Food? (Do you receive food stamps?)
    b. Clothing?

  c. Utilities?

  d. Other?

99. Is there anything you would like to change about your budget?

  a. If so, why?

100. How would you support yourself and child(ren) if you did not receive AFDC?

101. What effect does living on AFDC have on your child(ren)? On you?

102. What was it like for you to apply for AFDC?

103. What was the process like:

  a. How did you apply?

  b. What kind of paperwork was required?

  c. What kind of waiting period?

104. How old were you when you formed your own household?

105. What is your housing situation like?

  a. Do you have a roommate?

  b. How many rooms do you have?

  c. How often have you moved, and why?

106. Have you been denied housing for any reason?

107. How would you describe the quality of your life since you've been on AFDC?

108. What do you think about the AFDC policies?

109. Has your life changed in any way since you've been on AFDC?

SECTION 8. QUALITY OF LIFE

110. What were your plans before you had your first child and before you received AFDC?

111. What do you think about your lifestyle now?

112. What's your typical day like?

113. How would you describe the quality of your life since you've become a mother?

114. If on AFDC, how would you describe the quality of your life since you've been on AFDC?

115. Do you think your life is different from that of women who are not teenage mothers?

  a. If yes, why and how do you know this?

  b. If no, why not?

116. What do you think about friends and relatives who are on welfare?

117. Do you have teenage friends and relatives who are not on welfare?

  a. If yes, why aren't they on welfare?

  b. If no, how did they avoid it?

118. Do you think having children and being on welfare is a problem?

119. What kind of services does the welfare agency offer you?
120. What kind of program would you develop for women with children who need financial support?
121. If you lived your life over again, what would you change?
122. What would you leave as is?
123. Any suggestions for other women who may encounter similar experiences?

Now I would like to ask you what you thought about the interview questions:

124. What questions did you want me to ask you that I didn't ask?
125. What questions were helpful?
126. What questions were not helpful?

THANK YOU FOR THE INTERVIEW

Appendix C
Teen Mothers'
Demographic Characteristics

Name	Age	Age at Birth of First Child	Education	Source of Income	Family Origin Type†	Age of Mother at First Birth
Tracy Alexander	16	16	10th Grade	AFDC	F	16
Tonya Banks	26	18	High School Graduate	Employment	F	21
Annie Blake	18	15	Dropout	AFDC	F	23
Susan Carter°	16	15	Dropout	Mother	F	21
Jasmine Conners	17	16	10th Grade	Part-Time Employment	F	17
Denise Collins	25	18	High School Graduate	Employment	F	15
Alicia Cummins	26	17	Dropout	Employment	F	16
Junie Grant	15	14	9th Grade	Mother	F	24
Diane Harris°	20	17	Some College	AFDC	F	22
Carmilla Hopkins	16	15	Dropout	AFDC	F	22
Carita Hughes	20	15	Dropout	Employment	F	21
RoAnn James	18	17	High School Graduate	AFDC	TP	21
Evie Jenkins°	43	17	College Degree	Disability Insurance	TP	23
Lenora Jones	20	15	Dropout	Employment	TP	20
Shana Leeds°	17	16	Dropout	AFDC	F	22

Name						
LaShana Lewis	21	15	Dropout	AFDC	F	22
Dana Little	20	15	Dropout	AFDC	F	15
Irene Logan	21	18	Dropout	Unemployment Insurance	F	21
Melania Lowan	17	15	11th Grade	AFDC	TP	20
Jackie Marley	17	15	11th Grade	AFDC	F	15
Carolyn Mars	23	18	Dropout	Employment	TP	17
Marnie Martin	16	15	10th Grade	AFDC	TP	20
Roleta McMann	28	18	High School Graduate	AFDC	F	23
Georgia Minns	16	15	11th Grade	AFDC	F	15
Terry Parks°	18	16	Dropout	AFDC	F	16
Lois Patterson°	27	15	Dropout	AFDC	TP	15
Theresa Shimms	17	16	Dropout	Mother	F	15
DeLesha Simons	17	15	Dropout	Employment	TP	20
De Vonya Smalls°	16	15	12th Grade	AFDC	F	16
Margaret Thompson	40	15	Some College	Employment	F	21
Cassandra Witt	19	15	11th Grade	AFDC	F	16
Joanna Wright	35	18	College Degree	Employment	F	21

° Teen mothers who took part in participant observations and in-depth interviews.
† Family origin type: F = female-headed household; TP = two-parent household.

Notes

Introduction

1. See, for example, George Gilder, *Wealth and Poverty* (New York: Basic Books, 1983); Lawrence M. Mead, *Beyond Entitlement: The Social Obligations of Citizenship* (New York: Free Press, 1986); Daniel P. Moynihan, *Family and Nation: The Godkin Lectures at Harvard University* (San Diego: Harcourt Brace Jovanovich, 1987); Charles Murray, *Losing Ground: American Social Policy, 1950–1980* (New York: Basic Books, 1984). According to these authors, teenage mothers need moral character more than they need welfare benefits. Also see Charles Murray, "What Does the Government Owe the Poor? Conversation between Jesse Jackson and Charles Murray," *Harper's*, April 1986, pp. 35–39, 42–47.

2. In 1991 California ranked first in the percentage of first-born babies whose mothers were fifteen years and younger. California ranked fourth in births to Black teenage mothers under the age of twenty. See Kristin A. Moore, Angela Romano, and Cheryl Oakes, *Child Trends, Inc.* (Washington, D.C.: National Center for Health Statistics, Department of Health and Human Services, 1994). Also see James Trussell, "Teenage Pregnancy in the United States," in *Readings on Teenage Pregnancy from Family Planning Perspectives, 1985 through 1989* (New York: Alan Guttmacher Institute, 1990), 65; Oakland City Council, "Women and Children in Oakland" (September 1986); Karen Pittman, *Adolescent Pregnancy: An Anatomy of a Social Problem in Search of Comprehensive Solutions* (Washington, D.C.: Children's Defense Fund, 1987), 4; Karen Pittman and Gina Adams, *Teenage Pregnancy: An Advocate's Guide to the Numbers* (Washington, D.C.: Children's Defense Fund, 1988), 20. The notion of the underclass is certainly not new. Karl Marx described the lumpenproletariat a hundred years ago—the proletariat in rags, the very product of a capitalist society, the class composed

of people who had fallen through the cracks of society, "its human refuse." Marx meant to describe brawlers and street fighters in the service of rightist leaders like Napoleon III. In the 1960s Gunnar Myrdal used that idea to describe an emergent group composed mainly of young people who had been rendered superfluous and nonfunctional by economic development. The term *underclass* is currently used to describe people who engage in street crime and other forms of aberrant behavior and families with long-term spells of poverty or welfare dependency.

3. Alexis de Tocqueville, *Democracy in America*, ed. J. P. Meyer (New York: Doubleday, Anchor Books, 1969), 287.

4. Patricia Davis and Robert O'Harrow Jr., "The Hard Path from Welfare," *The Washington Post*, February 1994, 7–8. For examples of Black conservative thought, see Kevin Merida and Kenneth J. Cooper, "Black Lawmakers Sound the Alarm," *The Washington Post*, February 1994, 9. The authors made the point that some Black conservatives applauded a string of Supreme Court decisions that called into question race-conscious remedies for years of racial discrimination.

5. William J. Wilson, *The Truly Disadvantaged* (Chicago: University of Chicago Press, 1987).

Chapter 1

1. A. V. Richel, *Teen Pregnancy and Parenting* (New York: Hemisphere Publishing, 1989); Trussell, "Teenage Pregnancy," p. 66; Elaine Bell Kaplan, "Where Does a Fifteen-Year-Old Mother Turn?" *Feminist Issues* 8, no. 1 (spring 1988): 51–83. Also see Pittman and Adams, *Teenage Pregnancy*, p. 20. For discussion of the increasing numbers of Black teenage mothers, see Jaynes and Williams, *A Common Destiny;* Andrew M. Sum and W. Neal Fogg, "The Adolescent Poor and the Transition to Early Adulthood," in *Adolescence and Poverty: Challenges of the 1990s*, ed. Peter Edelman and Joyce Ladner (Washington, D.C.: Center for National Policy Press, 1991), 37–109.

2. See Moore, Romano, and Oakes, *Child Trends, Inc.* Also see *Statistical Abstract of the United States, 1994*, 114th ed. (Washington, D.C.: Bureau of the Census), table 71, p. 62; Nicholas Zill and Christine Winquist Nord, *Running in Place: How American Families Are Faring in a Changing Economy and an Individualistic Society* (Washington, D.C.: Child Trends, Inc., 1994).

3. Jaynes and Williams, *A Common Destiny*, p. 412; Moore, Romano, and Oakes, *Child Trends, Inc.* A high percentage of Black teenage mothers are giving birth to babies, but it is also true that Black teenage girls represent only 14 percent of all adolescent girls in the United States; therefore, the majority of teenage births are to White adolescent girls. Also see John Reid, "Blacks in America in the 1980s," *Population Bulletin* 37 (December 1982): 27; Chil-

dren's Defense Fund, *The Problems of Teenage Pregnancy, National Overview* (Washington, D.C.: Children's Defense Fund, 1988); S.L. Hofferth, J.R. Kahn, and W. Baldwin, "Premarital Sexual Activity among Teenage Women over the Past Three Decades," *Family Planning Perspectives* 19 (1988): 46.

4. Mead, *Beyond Entitlement;* Murray, "Conversation"; Gilder, *Wealth and Poverty;* Daniel Patrick Moynihan, *The Negro Family: The Case for National Action* (Washington, D.C.: U.S. Government Printing Office, 1965); Oscar Lewis, "The Culture of Poverty," *Scientific American* 215 (October 1966): 19–25.

5. Moynihan, *Negro Family.*

6. Patricia Hill Collins, *Black Feminist Thought* (New York: Routledge, 1991).

7. See R. W. Connell, *Gender and Power: The Person and Sexual Politics* (Stanford: Stanford University Press, 1987).

8. Peter Passell, "Economic Trends," *New York Times*, 20 June 1996, 2. Sheryl Stolberg, "Teen Pregnancies Force Town to Grow Up," *Los Angeles Times*, 29 November 1996, A56–A57.

9. Jaynes and Williams, *A Common Destiny*, p. 6; Sum and Fogg, "The Adolescent Poor"; Wilson, *The Truly Disadvantaged*, p. 3. For a perspective on Black teenage mothers different from Wilson's, see Arline Geronimus quoted in "Teenage Birth's New Conceptions," *Insight*, 30 April 1990, 12. Geronimus argues that for poor teenage girls with few opportunities, motherhood may be rewarding. The teen mothers in her study talk about motherhood in "positive terms." Geronimus claims that girls who have babies benefit in the long run because their children grow up while the mothers are still young, giving these mothers a better chance of getting on with their lives than those women who have children at a more traditional age. Geronimus's conclusions raise a number of questions: Did she read the literature on the consequences of early motherhood? Did she observe the teen mothers in their homes, or as they went about their daily lives? Did she ask questions that would penetrate the teen mothers' clever facades? If Geronimus had inquired further, we perhaps might have learned that the teenage girl who has her baby finds her life turned around, her social support system shaken, the baby's father vanished, and her character maligned.

10. Leon Dash, "Black Teenage Pregnancy in Washington D.C.," *International Social Science Review* 61 (autumn 1986): 4.

11. On the double standard, see Edwin Schur, *Labeling Women Deviant* (Philadelphia: Temple University Press, 1983), 83. Schur writes that a double standard exists regarding men's and women's sexual behavior. Women are much more likely than men to be seen as "fallen" when they fail to adhere to the social norms about out-of-wedlock pregnancy. A presumption is made about the character of the unwed mother but not about the unwed father. Schur states that there is "no popular imagery of the

unwed father." On the lack of information on sex and birth control, see
W.J. Lindermann and L. Scott, "Wanted and Unwanted Pregnancy in
Early Adolescence: Evidence from a Clinic Population," *Journal of Early
Adolescence* 1 (1983); E.A. Smith and J.R. Udry, "Coital and Non-Coital
Sexual Behaviors of White and Black Adolescents," *American Journal of
Public Health* 32 (1986): 234–256; C. Chilman, *Adolescent Sexuality in a
Changing Society*, 2d ed. (New York: Wiley, 1983); Christine Galavotti,
"Predictors of Risk-Taking, Preventive Behavior and Contraceptive Use
among Inner-City Adolescents" (Ph.D. diss., University of California,
Berkeley, 1987).

12. Carol Stack, *All Our Kin* (New York: Harper & Row, 1974), 62–89.

13. Stack, *All Our Kin*, p. 30.

14. Wilson, *The Truly Disadvantaged*, p. 176.

15. Carol Gilligan, Nona P. Lyons, and Trudy J. Hanmer, eds., *Making
Connections: The Relational Worlds of Adolescent Girls at Emma Willard
School* (Cambridge: Harvard University Press 1990); Robert Simmons and
Frances Rosenberg, "Disturbance in the Self-Image at Adolescence," *American Sociological Review* 38 (1973): 553–568.

16. Gilligan, Lyons, and Hanmer, *Making Connections*, p. 25.

17. See Althea Smith and Abigail J. Stewart, "Approaches to Studying
Racism and Sexism in Black Women's Lives," *Journal Of Social Issues* 39,
no. 3 (1983): 1–15; A. Brittany and Mary Maynard, *Sexism, Racism and Oppression* (New York: Basil Blackwell, 1984), 22. Collins, *Black Feminist
Thought*, p. 66. Collins makes the point that community structures resist
racial and class oppression. But gender crosses race and class structures and
provides fewer means of resistance.

18. Wilson, *The Truly Disadvantaged;* John Hope Franklin, "A Historical
Note on Black Families," in *Black Families*, 2d ed., ed. H.B. McAdoo (Newbury Park, Cal.: Sage Publications, 1988), 25–26. Also see Andrew Billingsley, *Climbing Jacob's Ladder* (New York: Simon & Schuster, 1992). Billingsley traces Black family structure from slavery to present.

19. Elijah Anderson, *Streetwise* (Chicago: University of Chicago Press,
1990), 73.

20. Erving Goffman, *Stigma* (Englewood Cliffs, N.J.: Prentice Hall,
1963), 23.

21. Wilson, *The Truly Disadvantaged*, p. 49. See Terry Williams and
William Kornblum, *Growing Up Poor* (Lexington, Mass.: Lexington Books,
1985), 3, for a description of the effect of economic changes on Black neighborhoods. Also see Jayne and Williams, *A Common Destiny*, p. 6; Raymond
S. Franklin, *Shadows of Race and Class* (Minneapolis: University of Minnesota Press, 1991); Barry Bluestone and Bennett Harrison, *The Industrialization of America* (New York: Harper & Row, 1982); Lawrence E. Gary, "A

Social Profile," in *Black Men,* ed. Lawrence E. Gary (Newbury Park, Cal.: Harper & Row, 1982), 29–45.

22. Williams and Kornblum, *Growing Up Poor,* pp. 3, 5. For other vivid portrayals of problems faced by inner-city children, see Alex Kotlowitz, *There Are No Children Here: The Story of Two Boys Growing Up in the Other America* (New York: Anchor Books, 1991); Jonathan Kozol, *Savage Inequalities: Children in America's Schools* (New York: Crown, 1991).

23. Richard B. Freeman and Harry J. Holzer, quoted in Jaynes and Williams, *A Common Destiny,* p. 320. Also see Ronald L. Taylor, "Black Youth in Crisis," in *The Black Family,* 5th ed., ed. Robert Staples (Belmont, Cal.: Wadworth, 1994), 214–229. Taylor argues that Black youth have become a "permanently entrapped population of poor persons largely isolated from the mainstream of American life" (214). Also see Williams and Kornblum, *Growing Up Poor,* p. 5. Williams and Kornblum write that changes in income may have a different psychological and cultural impact on Black adolescents than on White adolescents in industrial neighborhoods close to factories and other workplaces or on young people in "rural areas where work is plentiful even if jobs are scarce."

24. Williams and Kornblum, *Growing Up Poor;* Johnetta B. Cole, "Commonalities and Differences," in *All American Women: Lines That Divide, Ties That Bind,* ed. Johnetta B. Cole (New York: Free Press, 1986), 11.

25. Zill and Nord, *Running in Place,* p. 23.

26. Jaynes and Williams, *A Common Destiny,* p. 401. Also see "Percentage Comparison of African American and White Families Affected by Unemployment, 1988," *The State of Black America, 1990,* January 1990, p. 218.

27. Lawrence P. Crouchett, Lonnie G. Bunch III, and Martin Kendall Winnacker, *The History of the East Bay Afro-American Community, 1852–1977* (Oakland: Northern California Center for Afro-American History and Life, 1989), 21, 22.

28. Ibid. pp. 5, 9.

29. Ibid. pp. 10, 21, 22.

30. Ibid pp. 35, 41.

31. Ibid, p. 45.

32. Crouchett, Bunch, and Winnacker, *History,* p. 45; David Dante Troutt, *The Thin Red Line* (San Francisco: West Coast Regional Office, Consumers Union of the U.S., 1993).

33. Troutt, *Thin Red Line.*

34. See, for example, James Robbins, "Black Families: Identifying the Special Strengths—and Needs—of the Black Family," *Christian Science Monitor,* 16 May 1986, 2. See also Wilson, *The Truly Disadvantaged.*

35. See Troutt, *Thin Red Line.*

36. Ibid.

37. Claude Brown, "Return to Mean Streets," *Los Angeles Times*, 30 June 1986, 1B–2B.

38. Pearl Stewart, "Bleak Report on Oakland's Single Mothers," *San Francisco Chronicle*, 13 May 1986, 2.

39. Wilson, *The Truly Disadvantaged*. See report of Oakland City Council, "Women and Children of Oakland" (September 1986).

40. Oakland statistics from Oakland City Council, "Women and Children." Also see Pittman and Adams, *Teenage Pregnancy*, p. 20. On Richmond, see report released by Contra Costa County, "Contra Costa County Teen Pregnancy Statistics, 1986," pp. 1–3.

41. Twenty-three teen mothers said that they had little or no contact with their fathers; the remaining nine said that their fathers were "very supportive" or "somewhat" supportive. Twenty said they did not have much contact with the fathers of their babies. Other studies also report difficulties in interviewing teen mothers. For discussion, see Frank Furstenberg Jr., "Burdens and Benefits: Impact of Early Childbearing on the Family," *Journal of Social Issues* 36, no. 1 (1980): 123–135. Also see Karen Pittman and Gina Adams, *What about the Boys? Teenage Pregnancy Prevention Strategies* (Washington D.C.: Children's Defense Fund, 1988), p. 4. In reviewing strategies to increase babies' fathers' responsibilities to their children, Pittman and Adams note, "We need to start to talk to [fathers]." The Fund finds that teenage boys were primarily interested in discussing employment issues but not fatherhood issues.

42. For an overview of data on teenage pregnancies by age, see Trussell, "Teenage Pregnancy," pp. 65–75. Also see Wilson, *The Truly Disadvantaged;* Gerald D. Jaynes and Robin M. Williams, eds., *A Common Destiny: Blacks and American Society* (Washington, D.C.: National Academy Press, 1989), 401; Greg J. Duncan and Willard Rodgers, "Single-Parent Families: Are Their Economic Problems Transitory or Persistent?" *Family Planning Perspectives*, 19, no. 4 (July–August 1987): 171. Duncan and Rodgers examine the growth in the proportion of female-headed families from 1940 to the 1980s. My study is consistent with these studies on the sizable number of Black families in which both mother and daughter are teenage mothers.

43. See R. W. Connell's discussion of the social reproduction theory, *Gender and Power*. For an ethnographic treatment of Black women, see Joyce Ladner, *Tomorrow's Tomorrow: The Black Woman* (New York: Doubleday, 1970).

44. Ann Oakley first raised this issue in "Interviewing Women: A Contradiction in Terms," in *Doing Feminist Research*, ed. Helen Roberts (Boston: Routledge & Kegan Paul, 1981). Other sociologists have discussed the advantages or disadvantages of being inside or outside the culture being researched. See Alvin Gouldner, "Personal Reality and the Tragic Dimension

in Science," in *The Sociology of Research,* ed. G. Boalth (Carbondale: Southern Illinois University Press, 1969), 169–185; Ethel Sawyer, "Methodological Problems in Studying So-Called 'Deviant' Communities," in *The Death of White Sociology,* ed. Joyce Ladner (New York: Random House, 1973), 69; Oakley, "Interviewing Women." On rapport between an insider researcher and interviewees, see Gouldner, "Personal Reality."

45. On these issues faced by Black researchers studying the Black community, see Sawyer, "Methodological Problems," p. 69.

46. Nathan Hare and Julia Hare, *The Endangered Black Family* (San Francisco: Black Think Tank, 1984).

Chapter 2

1. David J. Dent, "The New Black Suburbs," *New York Times Magazine,* 14 June 1992, 22. Dent notes, "Middle-class blacks continue to follow their white counterparts to the suburbs." Between 1980 and 1990, the number of blacks living in the suburbs increased by 34 percent. Also see Karen DeWitt, "Wave of Suburban Growth Is Being Fed by Minorities," *New York Times,* 15 August 1994, A1, A12.

2. "Oakland School District," broadcast on radio station KPFA, Berkeley, 6 July 1991.

3. See Goffman, *Stigma.*

4. "Oakland School District." For discussion of problems facing Black students see Sylvia T. Johnson, "Extra-School Factors in Achievement, Attainment, and Aspirations among Junior and Senior High School-Aged Black Youth" (paper prepared for the Committee on the Status of Black Americans, National Research Council, Washington, D.C., 1987). Also see Roslyn A. Michelson and Stephen Samuel Smith, "Inner-City Social Dislocation and School Outcomes: A Structural Interpretation," in *Black Students,* ed. Gordon LaVern Berry and Joy Keiko Asamen (Newbury Park, Cal.: Sage Publications, 1989), 99–119; John Ogbu, *Minority Education and Caste* (New York: Academic Press, 1978). Ogbu reports that Black students find their culture in opposition to that of the school. See also Diane Scott-Jones, "Black Families and the Education of Black Children: Current Issues" (paper commissioned by the Committee on the Status of Black Americans, National Research Council, Washington, D.C., 1987), 81; William G. Spady, "The Impact of School Resources on Students," in *Review of Research in Education,* vol. 1, ed. Fred N. Kerlinger (Ithaca, Ill.: F.E. Peacock, 1993), 102–134. On family resources and academic performance, see Janice Hale-Benson, "The School Learning Environment and Academic Success," in Berry and Asamen, *Black Students,* p. 83. Also see Jacqueline Jordan Irvine, *Black Students and School Fail-*

ure: Policies, Practices, and Prescription (New York: Greenwood Press, 1990), 6.

5. Mark Snyder, "Self-Fulfilling Stereotypes," in *Racism and Sexism: An Integrated Study*, ed. Paula S. Rothenberg (New York: St. Martin's Press, 1988), 268. Snyder found that stigmatized people often believe the stereotypes about themselves. For similar ideas, see Michele Fine, "Sexuality, Schooling, and Adolescent Females: The Missing Discourse of Desire" *Harvard Educational Review* 58, no. 1 (February 1988): 64.

6. *National Center on Effective Secondary Schools Newsletter* (School of Education, University of Wisconsin–Madison) 4, no. 1 (spring 1989): 1. Also see William Lowes Boyd, "What Makes Ghetto Schools Work or Not Work?" (paper for conference "The Truly Disadvantaged," sponsored by the Social Science Research Council Committee for Research on the Urban Underclass and the Center for Urban Affairs and Policy Research, Northwestern University, Evanston, Ill., 19–21 October 1989), revised version (February 1990), 23; *National Center on Effective Secondary Schools Newsletter*, p. 4; Fine, "Adolescent Females"; Francis A. J. Ianni, *The Search for Structure: A Report on American Youth Today* (New York: Free Press, 1989), 143; R. C. Kessler and P.D. Cleary, "Social Class and Psychological Distress," *American Sociological Review* 45 (1980): 463–477. All of the authors argue that the life experiences of low-income Black teenagers bring about attitudes of distrust, fatalism, hostility, anti-intellectualism, apathy, hopelessness, and alienation.

7. Michele Fine, "Silencing in Public Schools," *Language Arts* 64 (1987): 157–174; "Adolescent Females," pp. 63–64. Fine writes, "expectations are often shaped unconsciously by the racist and sexist stereotypes that pervade our language" ("Adolescent Females," p. 64). Also see Paula S. Rothenberg, "The Prison of Race and Gender: Stereotypes, Ideology, Language, and Social Control," in Rothenberg, *Racism and Sexism*, p. 254. Rothenberg discusses ideology in explaining why people who live in the wealthiest country will not question why only the privileged enjoy a good education: "Instead of our being encouraged to ask why so much suffering and deprivation exist in the midst of such wealth, the prevailing racist and sexist ideology and stereotyping encourages us to redefine social problems as individuals' pathology." A good example of Rothenberg's point is California's governor Pete Wilson's use of the stereotype of lazy welfare recipients. Wilson remarked that he opposed welfare aid because he did not want to support people's beer habits. Also see Irvine, *Black Students and School Failure.* Irvine presents several examples of how Black teenage girls are ignored in school. When Black girls move from lower to upper elementary school grades, they begin to receive less and less feedback from their teachers and fewer opportunities to respond in class. They receive less positive feedback than other students. The lack of feedback

forces them to develop social rather than academic skills. In response they isolate themselves with other Black girls and work alone. They experience more negative interaction with teachers than other children do. Eventually, like Susan Carter, they become passive and invisible in the classroom.

8. See J. Brooks-Gunn and E. Reiter, "The Role of Pubertal Processes in the Early Adolescent Transition," in *The Developing Adolescent*, ed. S. Feldman and G. Elliot (Cambridge, Mass.: Harvard University Press, 1990), 24. Brooks-Gunn and Reiter write about adolescence as a stage at which the individual learns to form satisfying emotional attachments characterized by sensitivity, mutuality, responsibility, and trust. Also, adolescence is a difficult stage for most teenagers. Adolescents are beginning to confront school problems, identity problems, peer pressures, and developmental issues. Adolescents who, like many teen mothers I observed, do not receive adequate support, may become hesitant, passive, confused, submissive, and unlikely to have a sense of purpose. See Boyd, "Ghetto Schools." Boyd's study indicates that unsuccessful students respond to their plight in several ways, such as becoming hostile, swaggering, and making themselves appear street-wise.

9. Kozol, *Savage Inequalities*, p. 221. Kozol provides insightful observations. The public school system has become two-tiered: wealthy white students attend public schools that benefit from the fundraising efforts of their parents, and lower-income students do not have such wealth and as a result do not use the latest technological equipment or textbooks. Kozol says of the two-tiered California system: "In the affluent school districts, tax-exempt foundations have been formed to channel extra money into local schools. Afternoon 'Super Schools' have been created also in these districts to provide the local children with tutorials and private lessons. And 5 percent of California's public schools remain outside the 'spread' ($300) that exists between the other districts in official funding. The consequence is easily discerned by visitors. Beverly Hills still operates a high school that, in academic excellence, can rival those of Princeton and Winnetka. Baldwin Park still operates a poorly funded and inferior system. In Northern California, Oakland remains a mainly nonwhite, poor and troubled system while the schools that serve the Piedmont district, separately incorporated though it is surrounded on four sides by Oakland, remains richly funded, white and excellent. The range of district funding in the state is still extremely large. The poorest districts spend less than $3,000 while the wealthiest spend more than $7,000 [per student]." Also see Boyd, "Ghetto Schools."

10. See Hale-Benson, "School Learning Environment." Hale-Benson notes that Black families tend to encourage preadolescent girls to be self-sufficient since they are expected to eventually work. Preadolescent Black girls are likely to be more assertive and independent in a school setting than preadolescent white girls and tend to stay in school longer than Black boys. At schools these girls begin to find themselves being silenced.

11. Judith S. Musick, "The High-Stakes Challenge of Programs for Adolescent Mothers," in Edelman and Ladner, *Adolescence and Poverty,* pp. 111–137. According to Musick, childhood sexual victimization may leave a psychological residue of emotional discontinuity—a break between present and past, between thought and feeling, between actions and intentions—making the adolescent girl incline to both security-seeking behavior and security-threatening behavior.

12. Musick, "High-Stakes Challenge." Musick writes, "Teens told us their childhoods were filled with sexual abusive experiences that continued into early adolescence and beyond. Experiences were often coercive and sometimes aggressive, including rapes at knifepoint and boyfriends inviting their buddies to 'share' the frightened and confused victim." Also see John Briere, "The Long-term Clinical Correlates of Childhood Sexual Victimization" (paper presented at New York Academy of Science conference, New York, January 1987); Peter Blos, "The Child Analyst Looks at the Young Adolescent," in *Twelve to Sixteen: Early Adolescents*, ed. Jerome Kagan and Robert Coles (New York: W.W. Norton, 1972), 53.

13. See Brooks-Gunn and Reiter, "Role of Pubertal Processes," p. 24.

14. Private communication with Diane Russell, author of *The Secret Trauma: Incest in the Lives of Women* (New York: Basic Books, 1986). Russell was not surprised at the low number of reports of sexual abuse in my study. She suggests that statistics do not reveal the extent of the problem because many girls will not report sexual abuse. Also see Sharon Elise, "Teenage Mothers: A Sense of Self," in *African American Single Mothers: Understanding Their Lives and Families,* ed. Bette J. Dickerson (Thousand Oaks, Calif.: Sage Publications, 1995), 53–79. In Elise's study half of the twenty-four teenage mothers interviewed reported being sexually abused during early childhood. NBC's *Tom Brokaw Report* of 8 July 1992 finds that of three hundred high school girls interviewed, one out of four said that she had experienced some form of sexual abuse. Also see Hilary M. Lips, *Women, Men and Power* (London: Mayfield Publishing, 1991), 122–123. Lips contends that our double standard about sexual expectations and morality means that rape victims experience as much social rejection as rapists. One reason for the different standard is the attempt to pressure people to adhere to social norms. I talked to Millicent Robinson, a guidance counselor at an Oakland school. Millicent's concern for students had gained her the respect of many of the school's teenage mothers. Concerned about the numerous incidents of sexual abuse informally reported to her by teen mothers, she sent a questionnaire about sexual abuse to all of the school's 260 students, eighty of whom were teenage mothers. Twenty percent of the eighty teen mothers and 15 percent of those who were not teen mothers reported that they had been sexually abused by a relative, usually a stepfather, during early childhood.

15. The way the counselors handled this problem is similar to the way rape cases are handled: victims are often not believed or are perceived to be the one responsible for the abuse.

16. The fact that eating at fast-food restaurants was a favorite activity for many of the teen mothers means nothing until you examine what it tells you about inner-city life. See, for example, Alix M. Freedman, "Habit Forming, Fast-Food Chains Play a Central Role in Diet of the Inner-City Poor," *New York Times,* 19 December 1990, 1, 4. Freedman claims that fast-food chains like McDonald's are popular because they offer "affordable" food in a clean, safe, and comfortable place. He cites critics who believe that the proliferation of these stores means that "the underclass is held in a fast-food dietary prison, which produces nothing but bad health." Also see Troutt, *Thin Red Line.* One reason fast-food restaurants are so popular may be the difficulty of finding grocery stores. Troutt finds that the lack of large chain supermarkets in some Oakland neighborhoods makes food shopping more arduous than in middle-income communities. Very often, Oakland's low-income residents have to shop at the megastores and chain supermarkets in middle-income areas, such as those near Lake Merritt, the Diamond District, and Rockridge. They come as best they can—with children in tow, sometimes whole families, sometimes late at night or whenever else it is convenient.

17. Michele Wallace, *Black Macho and the Myth of the Super Woman* (New York: Dial Press, 1978), 80. Adolescents may face serious problems if their physical development makes them appear to be more mature than they are. See Blos, "Child Analyst," p. 53. He states, "The mastery of the world, concretely, symbolically, and conceptually, begins to serve as a self-regulatory source of self-esteem. And beyond that, it lifts the idiosyncratic childhood experiences onto the level of communicable and communal forms of expression." If we use Blos's theory in this case, it may mean that if teenage girls have not mastered their new identity, they may be confused by the sudden contradiction between their feelings and the way men and their families respond to them.

18. Quida E. Westney, Reness R. Jenkins, June Dobbs Butts, Irving Williams, "Dating and Sexual Patterns, Sexual Development and Behavior in Black Preadolescents," in *Young, Black and Male in America: An Endangered Species,* ed. Reginald Jones (Dover, Mass.: Auburn House Publishing, 1988), 55–65.

19. Ibid; Marie A. Vinovskis, "An 'Epidemic' of Adolescent Pregnancy? Some Historical Considerations," *Journal of Family History* 6, no. 2 (summer, 1981): 205–230; P. Reichelt and H. Werley, "Contraception, Abortion, and Venereal Disease: Teenagers' Knowledge and the Effect of Education," *Family Planning Perspectives* 7 (1975): 83–88; Kagan and Coles, *Twelve to Sixteen.*

20. Perhaps one way to change the cultural attitude about the menstrual cycle would be to institute a ritual celebrating menstruation and budding sexuality. Such a ritual would honor adolescence as a special time in a young girl's life. We could use as an example the Bat Mitzva celebration held for Jewish girls when they reach the age of thirteen. Another useful example is the Nevada Washoe Indians' celebration of their girls' passage to adulthood. They hold a dance in the young girl's honor along with a month-long celebration in which the girl, the center of attention and affection, is praised for making the passage into adulthood. Susan Carter said that she simply wanted her mother to say, "Congratulations, you're growing up."

21. See Greer Litton Fox and Judith K. Inazu, "Patterns and Outcomes of Mother-Daughter Communication about Sexuality," *Journal of Social Issues* 36, no. 1 (1980): 113. Also see Musick, "High-Stakes Challenge," p. 130.

22. There may be several reasons for Tracy's mother's failure to inform her daughter about birth control. She herself may be confused and uninformed about sexuality. See Ellen Eliason Kisker, "Teenagers Talk about Sex, Pregnancy and Contraception," *Family Planning Perspectives* 17, no. 2 (March–April 1985): 89. Kisker's study on adolescents' sexual behavior finds that parents are not better informed than their children. Several of the adult mothers in this study admitted they did not feel comfortable discussing sexual matters with their children. Also see Fox and Inazu, "Patterns and Outcomes," p. 9. The authors reviewed literature on parent and child communication about sexuality. They found that mothers of adolescents will not share actual information about their own sexual behavior. Although 76 percent of the mothers in the study were using birth control, their children reported that their mothers did not use any form of birth control. The authors found that children never cite parents as the source of information about sexuality. Also see Deborah Anne Dawson, "The Effects of Sex Education on Adolescent Behavior," *Family Planning Perspectives* 18, no. 4 (July–August 1986): 45–50; Joyce Ladner and Ruby Morton Gourdine, "Intergenerational Teenage Motherhood: Some Preliminary Findings," *Sage* (fall 1984): 22–24. Also see Barbara Ann Sachs, "The Relationship of Cognitive Development to Interpersonal Problem Solving Abilities in Female Adolescents" (Ph.D. diss., University of California, Berkeley, 1981). Sachs makes several excellent suggestions for informing inner-city adolescents: offer them contraceptive information, offer information at differing cognitive levels, develop and test tools to screen levels of cognitive development so that adolescents can be placed in different groups for developmentally based teaching, and help those who have chosen contraception to plan step-by-step means to reach their goal of nonreproduction. I would suggest, however, that before we can give them control over their reproductive behavior, they need to feel there is a reason to control it. Also see Christine Galavotti, "Predictors of Risk-Taking, Preventive

Behavior and Contraceptive Use among Inner-City Adolescents" (Ph.D. diss., University of California, Berkeley, 1987). Galavotti suggests that teenagers may not have a consistent view about control over health or pregnancy.

23. Elizah Anderson, "Sex Codes and Family Life among Poor Inner-City Youths," in *The Annals of the American Academy of Political and Social Science,* ed. William J. Wilson (Newbury Park, Cal.: Sage Publications, 1989), 59–78; Wallace, *Black Macho.*

24. See Sara McLanahan, "Family Structure and Stress: A Longitudinal Comparison of Two-Parent and Female-Headed Families," *Journal of Marriage and the Family* 9 (1983): 25. Also see G. Cvetknovitch and B. Grote, "Psychological Development and the Social Problem of Teenage Illegitimacy," in *Adolescent Pregnancy and Childbearing: Findings from Research,* ed. C. Chilman (Washington, D.C.: U.S. Department of Health and Human Services, 1980), 28; Robert Coles and Geoffrey Stokes, *Sex and the American Teenager* (New York: Harper & Row, 1985); M.L. Clark, "Friendships and Peer Relations of Black Adolescents," in *Black Adolescents,* ed. Reginald L. Jones (Berkeley: University of California Press, 1989), 174. Adolescents may be swayed to become sexually active by the belief that their friends are doing so.

25. Coles and Stokes, "Sex and the American Teenager." Cole and Stokes argue that other variables associated with socioeconomic status may also help explain the high rate of sexual activity among Black teenage males. For urban Black teenage males, poverty, poor educational facilities, high unemployment, fatalistic attitudes, and the need to "prove" oneself may play a significant role in early sexual experimentation. Private communication with Lillian Rubin, author of *Erotic Wars: What Happened to the Sexual Revolution?* (New York: Harper-Collins, 1990).

26. Anderson, "Sex Codes," pp. 59–78.

27. Dash, "Black Teenage Pregnancy," p. 9. Also see Judith Blake, *Comparative Youth Culture* (Boston: Routledge & Kegan Paul, 1985).

28. Kristen Luker, "Understanding the Risk-Taker," *The Family Planner* 30 (summer 1977): 1–2. Also see Kristen Luker, *Taking Chances: Abortion and the Decision Not to Contracept* (Berkeley: University of California Press, 1975); Judith Senderovitz and John M. Paxman, "Adolescent Fertility: Worldwide Concerns," *Population Bulletin* 40, no. 2 (April 1985): 22.

29. Alan Guttmacher Institute, *Fact Book on Teenage Pregnancy* (New York: Alan Guttmacher Institute, 1981). The Alan Guttmacher Institute reports that the general public supports sexuality education programs; however, the issue is controversial since opposition groups contend that information and education cause promiscuity.

30. See Susan Gustavus Philliber, "Socialization for Childbearing," *Journal of Social Issues* 36, no. 1 (1980): 230–245.

Chapter 3

1. The idea for separate schools was based on studies showing that teen mothers who complete high school do better financially than teen mothers who drop out of school. According to counselors at the Alternative Center, almost 20 percent of the students who attend alternative schools drop out each year. The others barely pass the standard tests for high school students. "The way the program works," a counselor told me, "is that these mothers attend classes three hours every morning where they take Math and English classes two hours and then attend parenting skills classes for an hour." The parenting skills hours were the most important, the counselor stressed, "because most teen mothers are so young and need to learn how to take care of their babies." The alternative schools (some teen mothers referred to them as "continuation" schools) also have a reputation as centers for juvenile delinquents. As one teen mother informed me, "You have to be either pregnant or you're not functioning well in regular school to go there."

2. The literature on teenage mothers also notes the high rates of infant morality and low birth weight of babies born to Black mothers. See Jaynes and Williams, *A Common Destiny*; Edelman and Ladner, *Adolescence and Poverty*.

3. Stack, *All Our Kin*.

4. Ibid.

5. Moynihan, *Negro Family*; Wilson, *The Truly Disadvantaged*.

6. Stack, *All Our Kin*; Herbert G. Gutman, *The Black Family in Slavery and Freedom, 1750–1925* (New York: Random House, 1976); Carl N. Degler, *At Odds: Women and the Family in America from the Revolution to the Present* (New York: Oxford University Press, 1980).

7. Billingsley, *Climbing Jacob's Ladder*; M. Belinda Tucker and Claudia Mitchell-Kernan, eds., *The Decline in Marriage among African Americans* (New York: Russell Sage Foundation, 1995); Stack, *All Our Kin*. Tucker and Mitchell-Kernan trace the changes in marriage rates and the socioeconomic problems faced by Black women and their children. They point out the need for studies on Black families that combine psychological perspectives with sociological, large aggregate, conceptualizations.

8. Pearl Stewart, "Guards at Apartments Give Up Their Shotguns," *San Francisco Chronicle*, 5 September 1987, 3.

9. Pearl Stewart, "Bleak Report on Oakland's Single Mothers," *San Francisco Chronicle*, 13 May 1986, 3; Shirley M.H. Hanson and Michael J. Sporokowski, "Single Parent Families," *Journal of Family Relations* 11 (January

1988): 3–8. Single-parent families headed by women have higher rates of poverty, higher minority representatives, and lower education than single-parent families headed by men.

Chapter 4

1. Gloria L. Joseph, "Mothers and Daughters: Traditional and New Perspectives," *Sage,* vol. 1, no. 2 (fall 1984); Nancy Chodorow, *The Reproduction of Mothering* (Berkeley: University of California Press, 1978); Nancy F. Russo, "The Motherhood Mandate," *Journal of Social Issues* 32 (1976): 143–153. Chodorow suggests that the relation between mother and daughter has a psychological base. She argues that separation in adolescence tends to be more difficult for daughters than for sons. Daughters never achieve a separate sense of self. She characterizes mothers' attitudes toward their adolescent daughters as "ambivalent" because the mothers want both to keep the daughters close and to push them into adulthood. According to Chodorow, women define themselves through their relationships with others. Daughters develop their identity as females by continuing their identification with their mothers. Chodorow's theory places girls and mothers into large categories on the basis of gender without discussing cultural and class differences.

2. Moynihan, *Negro Family;* Christopher Lasch, *Haven in a Heartless Land* (New York: Basic Books, 1972); Gilder, *Wealth and Poverty*, Murray, *Losing Ground*.

3. Most of this debate and scholarly discussion (including Chodorow's and Russo's) about the relationship between daughters and mothers has been written from a White middle-class perspective and assumes that all mothers are able to mother in the same way regardless of class or race. See, for example, Signe Hammer, *Mothers and Daughters/Daughters and Mothers* (New York: Quadrangle, 1975). Hammer examines the effect of racism on mother-daughter relationships. In seventy-five interviews with mothers and daughters from various ethnic backgrounds, she finds that racism has an impact on the ability of Black women to do good mothering. Despite the commonalities among all mothers, race and class differences affect the experiences of mothers.

4. This distinction is derived from the superb ethnography by Jay MacLeod, *Ain't No Makin' It: Leveled Aspirations in a Low-Income Neighborhood* (Boulder: Westview Press, 1987).

5. Since the uncle who had sexually abused Susan was still living with her grandmother, Susan was not sure how much she could trust her grandmother to support her.

6. Patricia Hill Collins, "The Meaning of Motherhood in Black Culture and Black Mother/Daughter Relationships," *Sage,* 4 (fall 1987): 3–10.

7. See Ladner and Gourdine, "Intergenerational Teenage Motherhood," p. 23.

8. Ibid.

9. See LaRue Allen and David W. Britt, "Black Women in American Society: A Resource Development Perspective," in *Social Psychological Problems of Women: Prevention and Crisis Invention*, ed. Annette G. Richel, Meg Gerrard, and Ira Iscoe (New York: Hemisphere Publication, 1984), 74. Also see Richard E. Ball, "Marital Status, Household Structure, and Life Satisfaction of Black Women," *Social Problems* 20 (April 1983); Cynthia Costello and Anne J. Stone, eds., *The American Woman, 1994–95* (New York: W.W. Norton, 1994), 119. According to Costello and Stone, depression rates among teenage girls have increased in recent years.

10. Goffman, *Stigma*, p. 63.

11. See Bell Kaplan, "Women's Perceptions of the Adolescent Experience," *Adolescence* (in press). Kaplan studies racially and ethnically diverse groups of middle-class women undergraduate students who find that negative experiences during early adolescence continue to haunt them in their adult years.

12. Furstenberg, "Burdens and Benefits," p. 230.

13. Schur, *Labeling Women Deviant*.

14. Dennis P. Hogan and Evelyn M. Kitagawa, "The Impact of Social Status, Family Structure, and Neighborhood on the Fertility of Black Adolescents," *American Journal of Sociology* 90 (1985): 831; Linda M. Burton and Vern L. Bengtson, "Black Grandmothers: Issues of Timing and Continuity of Roles," in *Grandparenthood*, ed. Vern Bengtson and J. Robertson (Beverly Hills: Sage Publications, 1985), 75. Hogan and Kitagawa's study of teen mothers and Burton and Bengtson's descriptions of "off-time" mothers match many of my own observations of the teen mothers' and adult mothers' lives. Hogan and Kitagawa suggest that Black teenagers who reside in female-headed households in "high risk social environments" (such as Oakland and Richmond) face circumstances, such as poverty and unstable family life, that increase their chances of becoming teenage mothers. In a study of mothers who have teenage daughters, Burton and Bengtson find that "the off-time accession to the lineage role creates," for many young mothers, tensions and conflicts in their views of themselves and in their families' systems of cohesion and social support. Burton and Bengtson find that women who assume the grandmother role "off time" may experience "crisis accumulation." The authors cite the case of a twenty-seven-year-old mother of a teenage mother who had to assume the grandparent/surrogate parent role when her daughter was unable to care for the new baby. But she also had a small child of her own. According to the authors, parenting and grandparenting demands, coupled with those of work and from other generational

family members, make the grandmother vulnerable to "role overload." The role overload is "potentially catastrophic." The grandmother's daughter had difficulty responding to her role as mother because she wanted to do "teenage things." The grandmother did not engage in grandparenting behavior because she felt that it made her look "old." "Off-time" grandmothering roles created tensions and conflicts in the family. Both Hogan and Kitagawa and Burton and Bengtson offer only a superficial view of these Black adult and teen mothers. Also see Richie Solinger, *Wake Up Little Susie: Single Pregnancy and Race before Roe v. Wade* (New York: Routledge, 1992).

15. Maxine Baca Zinn, "Family, Race, and Poverty in the Eighties," *Signs: Journal of Women in Culture and Society* 14 (1989): 189–218.

16. Ladner and Gourdine, "Intergenerational Teenage Motherhood."

17. Robert Staples, "Changes in Black Family Structure: The Conflict between Family Ideology and Structural Conditions," *Journal of Marriage and the Family* 47 (November 1985): 1005–1013. Staples quotes several studies indicating that Blacks tend to be religious, to believe in hard work, and to be strongly supportive of family life. Staples suggests that Blacks tend to be liberal on social and economic policies, but hold traditional, "even conservative," attitudes on moral issues. Staples concludes that although "Black women state that they wish to marry and maintain traditional roles in the conjugal relationship," studies showing the decline of marriage rates among Blacks reflect the gap between the mainstream ideology of lower- and middle-income Blacks and "the reality in which [Blacks] live their lives" (p. 1011).

18. Stack, *All Our Kin*.

19. Lucy Rose Fischer, *Linked Lives: Adult Daughters and Their Mothers* (New York: Harper & Row, 1987), 20.

Chapter 5

1. Shirley Foster Hartley, *Illegitimacy* (Berkeley: University of California Press, 1983), 2. The major task for Terry had to do with what Hartley referred to as the "assignment" of the father. The unwed mother has to hope that the baby's father is committed to her and the baby. If there is any doubt in his mind or if other issues arise, he may simply walk away. Hartley writes, "Since the female is biologically tied to the child, through the period of pregnancy and lactation, it is her period of maximum dependency, as well as a time of complete helplessness for the infant." Harley quotes research on unwed mothers to show that women who are alone and "lacking a secure commitment on the part of the child's father" lack self-esteem. Furthermore, Hartley believes that even where financial support is not a problem, the emotional warmth, security, and consistency so important in child rearing "may be missing when the father is not available."

2. Jewelle Taylor Gibbs, "Conclusions and Recommendations," in *Young Black and Male in America,* ed. Jewelle Taylor Gibbs (Dover, Mass.: Auburn House, 1988), 342. Gibbs finds that low-income youth have negative attitudes toward conceptions.

3. Carlo Salguero, "The Role of Ethnic Factors in Adolescent Pregnancy and Motherhood," in *Adolescent Parenthood,* ed. Max Sugar (New York: Spectrum Publications, 1984), 81–95. Also see James M. Herzog's study, "Boys Who Make Babies," in *Adolescent Parenthood,* pp. 96–112; Pittman and Adams, "What about the Boys?"; Hartley, *Illegitimacy,* p. 13.

4. Hartley, *Illegitimacy,* p. 13.

5. *Essence,* August–September 1987, 10–11.

6. Carol Gilligan, *In a Different Voice* (Cambridge, Mass: Harvard University Press, 1987). We can put the idea of boys learning to devalue girls at an early age alongside studies indicating that although these teen mothers lived in the same neighborhood and were nearly the same age as the teen fathers, they lived in quite different—and gendered—worlds. See, for example, Lawrence E. Gary, "Predicting Interpersonal Conflict between Men and Women: The Case of Men," in *Changing Men: New Directions in Research on Men and Masculinity,* ed. Michael S. Kimmel (Newbury Park, Cal.: Sage Publications, 1987), 232–243. Gary makes the point that social life in the community is gender segregated. Although Gary does discuss teenage fathers, his observations provide insight regarding how these men might be socialized about relationships and commitment. The men in Gary's study spent more time with work colleagues, with male friends in bars, and at sporting activities. The women spent more time with relatives, children, and women friends. They seldom shared activities. As one might expect, the lack of interaction seems to produce in these men little idea—or understanding—of the importance of companionship and commitment in couple relationships. Gary believes that these problems are a major source of tension between the women and men in his study. Since the tension created by the gendered world Gary observes couples with the idea that men are more highly valued in this society than women, these men may not learn to care for women. Gary's studies of men's segregated lives, and the teen mothers' observations, suggest that these men's lives are structured in such a male-centered way that, as I suspect and as Gary suggests, they would not learn to interact with women other than in sexual relations. Also see Douglas Glasgow, *The Underclass: Poverty, Unemployment, and Entrapment of Ghetto Youth* (San Francisco: Jossey-Bass Publishers, 1980). In Glasgow's study the men felt left out of the economic structure and felt their "manhood" affected because they could not be breadwinners, and they demonstrated their masculinity by finding "alternatives" such as sexual conquest. Since they felt cheated by society and did not believe women to be their equals, they developed a "streetmen's

ideology" that said women are supposed to be sexually exploited. To these men, having "sex and children" establishes their masculinity when work does not.

Also see Andrew Tolson, *The Limits of Masculinity* (New York: Harper & Row, 1977), 60. Tolson points to the dysfunctional aspect of masculinity traits such as toughness, aggressiveness, and dominance. These traits are manifested by men who restrict social relationships to men and see women primarily as sexual partners. A banding together against women unites the individuals into the collective of the work group and the company of men. They gloss over the contradictions of male chauvinism and laugh off the unease that men feel about their need for love and the support of women. Tolson adds, "Unhappily, this often takes the form of needing women for sexual and domestic services, but saving their deeper feelings for other men with whom there is no complication of sexual relations." Also see Gregory M. Herek, "On Heterosexual Masculinity: Some Psychical Consequences of the Social Construction of Gender and Sexuality," in Kimmel, *Changing Men*, p. 72. According to Herek, heterosexual masculinity embodies personal characteristics such as "success and status, toughness and independence, aggressiveness and dominance." Adult men manifest these aggressive tendencies through exclusively social relationships with men and primarily sexual relationships with women. Since being masculine is defined by these characteristics, being a man "requires not being compliant, dependent, or submissive; not being effeminate (a 'sissy') in physical appearance or mannerism; not having relationships with men that are sexual or overly intimate and not failing in sexual relationships with women."

7. Jessie Bernard, "The Good Provider Role: Its Rise and Fall," in *Family in Transition*, ed. Arlene S. Skolnick and Jerome Skolnick (Boston: Little, Brown, 1986), 125–144. See Wilson, *The Truly Disadvantaged;* Glasgow, *Underclass;* Jaynes and Williams, *A Common Destiny;* Elliot Liebow, *Tally's Corner* (Boston: Little, Brown, 1975); Robert Staples, *Masculinity* (San Francisco: Scholar Press, 1982).

8. Wilson, *The Truly Disadvantaged*.

9. Staples, *Masculinity*, p. 27.

10. Troy Duster, "Social Implications of the 'New' Urban Underclass," (unpublished paper, 1984); Jaynes and Williams, *A Common Destiny;* Daniel Thompson, *The Sociology of the Family* (New York: Dial Press, 1980), 10. Also see Wilson, *The Truly Disadvantaged;* Glasgow, *Underclass;* Liebow, *Tally's Corner;* Staples, *Masculinity*.

11. Laurie Davidson and Laura Kramer Gordon, *The Sociology of Gender* (Chicago: Rand McNally College Publishing, 1979).

12. Anderson, *Streetwise*, p. 117.

13. Anderson, *Streetwise*.

14. Ibid.

15. Noel Cazanave, "Men in America: The Quest for Manhood," in *Black Families*, 1st ed., ed. Harriet Pipes McAdoo (Beverly Hills: Sage Publications, 1981), 35.

16. Anderson, *Streetwise,* p. 133.

17. Josephina J. Card and Lauress L. Wise, "Teenage Mothers and Teenage Fathers: The Impact of Early Childbearing on the Parents' Personal and Professional Lives," in *Teenage Sexuality, Pregnancy, and Childbearing,* ed. Frank F. Furstenberg Jr., Richard Lincoln, and Jane Menken (Philadelphia: University of Pennsylvania Press, 1981), 211–222.

18. Anderson, *Streetwise,* p. 133. Also see Marcia Guttentag and Paul F. Secord, *Too Many Women? The Sex Ratio Question* (Beverly Hills: Sage Publications, 1983), 228. Guttentag and Secord gathered a variety of data based on studies of the low sex ratio of the Black community to conclude that the large pool of available women means that men are more likely to devalue marriage, less likely to commit to relationships, and less inclined to feel the need to marry. The authors quote one observer of the community who contends, "An appropriate analog is witnessed every day in the American market place. As the availability of a commodity decreases and the need for that commodity increases the price will invariably climb." In one sense, men may be viewed as a commodity in short supply and high demand: "Where women are plentiful, they are likely to tolerate certain abuses because of lack of alternatives." The authors also cited one survey indicating that far more teenage girls than boys hoped to be married some day. See Tucker and Mitchell-Kernan, *Decline in Marriage among African Americans,* p. 346. In this comprehensive study of the socioeconomic factors that lead to declining rates of marriage among Black women, the authors link the low sex ratio to premarital childbirth: "A very strong negative relationship between sex ratios and nonmarital births—that is, fewer men relative to women—was associated with an increase in births outside of marriage."

19. California may have a dual civil-criminal system of family law. According to Charlene Simmons, "Custodial vs. Non-Custodial Parents: A Case Study of Family Support Division, Sacramento County, California" (Ph.D. diss., University of California, Berkeley, 1986), middle-class divorced noncustodial parents received civil enforcement, and low-income noncustodial parents, especially welfare families, received criminal enforcement, with its harsher procedures and penalties. Since four-fifths of the families in the sample received AFDC, and over half were informally separated, criminal law is the agency's primary child support mechanism—a reality missed by studies restricted to divorce samples. The impoverished noncustodial fathers of welfare families are cited for nonsupport and incarcerated more often, while

wealthier parents have their incomes attached. Bureaucracies administer laws requiring the absence of the principal wage-earning parent for AFDC eligibility, and then prosecute that parent for nonsupport, thereby criminalizing the relationships of impoverished families.

Chapter 6

1. Linda Leonard, *The Wounded Woman* (Athens: Ohio University Press, Swallow Press, 1982), 23.

2. Fischer, *Linked Lives*, p. 3.

3. Goffman, *Stigma.*

4. See Jack W. Sattel, "Men, Inexpressiveness, and Power," in *Feminist Frontiers,* ed. Laurel Richardson and Verta Taylor (New York: Random House, 1986).

5. Arlie Russell Hochschild suggested this emotion management strategy in a personal communication.

6. Her choice is interesting because the series originally appeared on television in the 1970s, a time of newly working White mothers. But the series' emphasis on breadwinner dad and housewife mom was a throwback to the 1950s' patriarchal *Father Knows Best* television family.

7. James L. Caughey, *Imaginary Social Worlds* (Lincoln: University of Nebraska Press, 1984), 40, 54.

8. For an example of this thinking, see Ron Cortes, "The $10 Million Teenage Director," *The Philadelphia Inquirer,* 3 July 1990, 20–21. The article quotes an interview with Matty Rich, a nineteen-year-old teenager who gained a measure of fame for directing a successful movie, *Straight out of Brooklyn,* about a hard-drinking and frustrated father like his own. The interviewer asked Matty Rich what inspired him. "The first thing that inspired me was the Brady Bunch. When Peter spilled ice cream all over the floor, Mr. Brady was nice about it. But when I spilled ice cream on the floor, I got slapped. I kept wondering why my father wasn't like Mr. Brady."

9. Musick, "High-Stakes Challenge," pp. 118–153.

10. A recent television commercial—its product geared it to parents of teenagers—depicted a White teenage girl getting ready for her first date. By 1990s dress standards she looked rather prim, in a high-neck dress and a pink hair bow. Her mother and father beamed when the date guided her out of the door, after, of course, Dad planted a kiss on his daughter's cheeks. If one could speculate about the life chances of this young girl, given her middle-class situation, most likely she will date for a while, then marry during her early to middle twenties. After a decent interval, say, several years, she will have two children. Then she will retire to the family home to raise the children. If she is "a nineties woman," at some point she may find low-

income employment. Her first priority, however, will be the family. When we look at the television image again, we find that this adolescent girl image rarely fits the realities of most Black teenage girls.

11. Bernard, *Good Provider Role.*

12. See Judith Blake, *Family Structure in Jamaica* (New York: Free Press of Glencoe, 1985). Blake finds similar issues of status transmission in her study of Black families in Jamaica.

13. Anderson, *Streetwise,* p. 9.

14. Ibid.

15. See A.F. Welbourne, "The Relation of Parental Sexual Knowledge and Attitudes and Communication about Sexual Topics with Their Early Adolescent Children" (Ph.D. diss., New York University, 1977), p. 41. The study finds substantial evidence that many families prefer male children to female children.

16. See Warren B. Miller, "Psychological Vulnerability to Unwanted Pregnancy," in Furstenberg, Lincoln, and Menken, *Teenage Sexuality,* p. 352.

17. C. Wright Mills, *The Sociological Imagination* (New York: Oxford University Press, 1959), 5.

Chapter 7

1. Moore, Romano, and Oakes, *Child Trends, Inc.*

2. David T. Ellwood, *Poor Support: Poverty in the American Family* (New York: Basic Books, 1988), 168. Ellwood examines welfare policies and offers guidelines for changing child support. "[If we do] three things—identify both parents at the birth of a child, move to a uniform system of payments based on the income of the absent parent, and have employers collect all payments automatically—we would go a long way toward improving the situation of children in single-parent homes" (p. 164). Ellwood's suggestions may alleviate a few of these children's problems, but nothing short of major economic changes that center on giving poor mothers (and other poor families) stable jobs with good wages will solve the economic plight of these children.

3. Lar A. Levitan, *Program in Aid of the Poor,* 8th ed. (Baltimore: Johns Hopkins University Press, 1981.) Also see Jaynes and Williams, *A Common Destiny.* Jaynes and Williams find that family assistance programs such as AFDC do not abolish poverty for children. For studies on family assistance programs, see David Ellwood and Lawrence H. Summers, "Poverty in America: Is Welfare the Answer or the Problem?" in *Fighting Poverty: What Works and What Doesn't,* ed. Sheldon H. Danzinger and Daniel H. Weinberg (Cambridge, Mass: Harvard University Press, 1986), 33–65; Irwin Garfinkel and Sara S. McLanahan, *Single Mothers and Their Children: A*

New American Dilemma (Washington, D.C.: Urban Institute, 1986); H. L. Ross and I. Sawhill, *Time of Transition: The Growth of Families Headed by Women* (Washington, D.C.: Urban Institute, 1975); Kristin Moore and Martha R. Burt, *Private Crisis, Public Cost: Policy Perspectives on Teenage Childbearing* (Washington, D.C.: Urban Institute, 1982).

4. Levitan, *Program in Aid*. See Irene Diamond, ed., *Introduction to Families, Politics, and Public Policy* (New York: Longman, 1983). For an assessment of studies on family assistance benefits, see Jaynes and Williams, *A Common Destiny*, pp. 531–533. For an overview of the policies of the 1960s, see Frances Fox Piven and Richard A. Cloward, *Regulating the Poor: The Function of Public Welfare* (New York: Vintage Books, 1993). See Morris Janowitz, *Social Control of the Welfare State* (Chicago: University of Chicago Press, 1976).

5. Moynihan, *Negro Family*, p. 5.

6. Michael Harrington, *The New American Poverty* (New York: Penguin Books, 1986). Also see Diane Pearce, "The Feminization of Ghetto Poverty," *Society* 5 (November–December 1983): 24–27; Jaynes and Williams, *A Common Destiny*.

7. Harrington, *New American Poverty*.

8. Ibid., p. 5; Pearce, "Feminization of Ghetto Poverty"; Jayne and Williams, *A Common Destiny*.

9. Robert L. Allen, *Black Awakening in Capitalist America* (Garden City, N.Y.: Doubleday Anchor Books, 1969), 25; Sara Evans, *Personal Politics* (New York: Vintage Books, 1979); David Whitman, "Liberal Rhetoric and the Welfare Underclass," *Society* 24 (November–December 1983): 12; Harrington, *New American Poverty*.

10. Wilson, *The Truly Disadvantaged*, p. 29. Also see Ruth Sidel, *Women and Children Last* (New York: Viking Penguin, 1986).

11. Margaret L. Anderson, *Thinking about Women*, 2d ed. (New York: Macmillan, 1983). Also see bell hooks, *Ain't I a Woman?* (Boston: South End Press, 1981); Imelda Whelehan, *Modern Feminist Thought: From the Second Wave to "Post-Feminism"* (New York: New York University Press, 1995).

12. One social worker, who described herself as jaded and fed up, was very critical of the social service agency where she had worked for twenty years. I asked her about the teen mothers' reports that their papers did not reach the workers and that rude workers seemed to intentionally delay the process by refusing to meet with the teen mothers or return their telephone calls. She responded: "If the workers don't like you, they can lose the papers, ask a lot of irrelevant questions, or be sullen in their interaction with you." As she saw it, "the workers have some power in slowing down the procedure if they think for any reason that the recipient doesn't deserve the welfare aid."

13. Joseph Rogers, "Fighting Back: Nine Modes of Adaptation of a Deviant Label," *Social Problems* 33, no. 3 (January–February 1982): 111–123.

14. Ibid.

15. See Fox and Inazu, "Patterns and Outcomes"; Nancy Folbre, "The Pauperization of Motherhood: Patriarchy and Public Policy in the United States," *Review of Radical Political Economics* 16, no. 4 (winter 1984): 12; Elise F. Jones et al., *Teenage Pregnancy in Industrial Countries* (New Haven, Conn.: Yale University Press, 1986). The act was passed, in large part because it promised to reduce net expenditures of AFDC. In 1984 both the House of Representatives and the Senate approved a bill that would require states to withhold money from the paychecks of parents in arrears on child support payments. This law is only effective if the father can be located.

16. Goffman, *Stigma,* p. 63.

17. A number of studies have been unable to confirm the question of whether differential welfare payments encourage adolescent pregnancy. See Jones et al., *Teenage Pregnancy in Industrial Countries;* Philip Cutwright, "Illegitimacy and Income Supplements" in *Studies in Public Welfare,* paper 12, pt. I, 90, Joint Economic Committee of the Congress, ed. R. Lerman and A. Townsend (Washington, D.C.: U.S. Government Printing Office, 1973); Kristin A. Moore, "The Effect of Government Policies on Out-of-Wedlock Sex and Pregnancy," *Family Planning Perspectives* 9 (1977): 16; Paul J. Placek and Gerry E. Hendershot, "Public Welfare and Family Planning: An Empirical Study of the Brood Sow Myth," *Social Problems* 23 (1975): 226. Yet some authors continue to make this argument. See Victor Fuchs, *How We Live: Economic Perspectives on Americans from Birth to Death* (Cambridge, Mass.: Harvard University Press, 1983); Murray, *Losing Ground;* Jane Sklar and Beth Berkow, "Teenage Family Formation in Postwar America," *Family Planning Perspectives* 6 (1974): 80.

18. See G. J. Duncan and Willard Rodgers, "Single-Parent Families: Are Their Economic Problems Transitory or Persistent?" *Family Planning Perspectives* 19, no. 4 (July–August 1987): 50–55.

19. See Frank Furstenberg Jr. and Albert G. Crawford, "Family Support: Helping Teenage Mothers to Cope," in Furstenberg, Lincoln, and Menken, *Teenage Sexuality,* pp. 280–320; Kristin A. Moore and Steve B. Caldwell, "The Effect of Government Policies on Out-of-Wedlock Sex and Pregnancy," in Furstenberg, Lincoln, and Menken, *Teenage Sexuality,* pp. 126–135. Also see Jaynes and Williams, *A Common Destiny,* p. 290. According to Jaynes and Williams, a 1987 report from the U.S. House of Representatives Committee on Ways and Means shows that a woman working full time at a five-dollars-per-hour job (and thus earning ten thousand dollars in gross pay annually) will have only $1,500 more in disposable income

than from family assistance benefits, and she will have lost her government medical protection (Medicaid).

20. Furstenberg and Crawford, "Family Support."

21. See Paula Ries and Anne J. Stone, eds., *The American Woman, 1992–93: A Status Report* (New York: W.W. Norton, 1992).

22. Gary A. Tobin, ed., *Divided Neighborhoods: Changing Patterns of Racial Segregation* (Newbury Park, Cal.: Sage Publications, 1987), 12.

23. Goffman, *Stigma;* Laud Humphreys, *Tearoom Trade: Impersonal Sex in Public Places*, 2d. ed., (Chicago: Aldine, 1975), 139–140.

24. Goffman, *Stigma.*

25. Arlie Russell Hochschild, "The Sociology of Feeling and Emotions: Selected Possibilities," in *Another Voice*, ed. Marcia Millman (New York: Anchor Books, 1975), 219.

26. For a discussion of the doublemindedness of America, see Lewis Lapham, *Money and Class in America* (New York: Ballantine Books, 1988). The author makes the point that on the one hand, America preaches equality for all, while on the other hand, there are social problems that must be overcome if equality is to be possible.

27. Mark Robert Rank, *Living on the Edge: The Realities of Welfare in America* (New York: Columbia University Press, 1994), 30.

Chapter 8

1. Erving Goffman, *Frame Analysis* (New York: Harper & Row, 1974).

2. Rogers, "Fighting Back."

3. Elizabeth Rauh Bethel, *Promiseland: A Century of Life in a Negro Community* (Philadelphia: Temple University Press, 1981), 157. Also see Gutman, *Black Family*, p. 25. Herbert Gutman made an observation similar to Bethel's in his study of a Black community in rural Alabama in the 1920s. That community referred to children born out of wedlock as "outside" children. Although those families did not condemn the mothers of these children, Gutman found that the church "[tended to frown upon] sexual irregularity and applied social pressure toward sexual morality by barring offenders from church until they repented."

4. Phyliss Evelyn Morgan, "The Church of God Minister's Perception of Unwed, Teenage Pregnancy in the Church and Community" (Ph.D. diss., University of California, Berkeley, 1985). The conservative mindset of the church is shown by Phyllis Morgan's interviews with Black ministers. She asked ministers to discuss their views on the high rate of teenage pregnancy in their communities. The ministers placed emphasis on the failure of the parents to instill the right kind of moral value in their children as the primary influence leading to teenage pregnancy. See Billingsley, *Climbing Jacob's*

Ladder. Billingsley presents an overview of Black churches' social and political influence in the Black community and the larger society.

5. Goffman, *Stigma,* p. 42.

6. I also suspect that the counselors wanted the teen mothers to verify their need for the teen parent program. If the teen mothers said they were not making progress in getting their lives together, the counselors could request additional aid. Even in this case it was unlikely that their request would be honored by the parent organization, because the Reagan administration had cut back on funding social service agencies.

7. Goffman, *Stigma,* pp. 42, 57.

8. See Jaynes and Williams, *A Common Destiny.*

Chapter 9

1. Moynihan, *Negro Family;* Wilson, *The Truly Disadvantaged;* Stack, *All Our Kin.*

2. Quoted in Wilson, *The Truly Disadvantaged,* pp. 73–74.

3. Gilligan, Lyons, and Hanmer, *Making Connections.*

4. David L. Morgan, "Strategies and Sociologists: A Comment on Crow," *Sociology* 23, (1989): 25–29.

5. Fischer, *Linked Lives.*

6. Mary McGrory, "What to Do about Parents of Illegitimate Children," *The Washington Post,* 15 February 1994, 25.

7. Kristen Luker, *Deceptive Conceptions* (Cambridge, Mass.: Harvard University Press, 1996); Ruth Horowitz, *Teen Mothers: Citizens or Dependents* (Chicago: University of Chicago Press, 1995); Judith S. Musick, *Young, Poor, and Pregnant: The Psychology of Teenage Motherhood* (New Haven, Conn.: Yale University Press, 1993).

Appendix A

1. Anselm L. Strauss, *Qualitative Analysis for Social Science* (New York: Cambridge University Press, 1987); Oakley, "Interviewing Women"; Shulamit Reinhartz, *On Becoming a Social Scientist: From Survey Research and Participant Observation to Experiential Analysis* (San Francisco: Jossey-Bass, 1979).

2. Strauss, *Qualitative Analysis*, p. 65.

3. Oakley, "Interviewing Women," p. 25.

4. Reinhartz, *Becoming a Social Scientist*, p. 28.

5. Troy Duster, "Diversity and Multiculturalism in Higher Education: Can We Elevate the Dialog and Address the Experience?" speech at University of Southern Calfornia, 30 November 1992.

6. Norman Denzin, "On the Ethics of Disguised Observation," *Social Problems* 15 (1968): 502–504.

Bibliography

Alan Guttmacher Institute. *Fact Book on Teenage Pregnancy.* New York: Alan Guttmacher Institute, 1981.

Allen, LaRue, and David W. Britt. "Black Women in American Society: A Resource Development Perspective." In *Social Psychological Problems of Women Prevention and Crisis Invention,* edited by Annette G. Richel, Meg Gerrard, and Ira Iscoe. New York: Hemisphere Publishing, 1984.

Allen, Robert L. *Black Awakening in Capitalist America.* Garden City, N.Y.: Doubleday Anchor Books, 1969.

Anderson, Elijah. "Sex Codes and Family Life among Poor Inner-City Youths." In *The Annals of the American Academy of Political and Social Science,* edited by William J. Wilson. Newbury Park, Calif.: Sage Publications, 1989.

———. *Streetwise.* Chicago: University of Chicago Press, 1990.

Anderson, Margaret L. *Thinking about Women,* 2d ed. New York: Macmillan, 1983.

Baca Zinn, Maxine. "Family, Race, and Poverty in the Eighties." *Signs: Journal of Women in Culture and Society* 14 (1989): 189–218.

Ball, Richard E. "Marital Status, Household Structure, and Life Satisfaction of Black Women." *Social Problems* 20 (April 1983): 22.

Bernard, Jessie. "The Good Provider Role: Its Rise and Fall." In *Family in Transition,* edited by Arlene S. Skolnick and Jerome Skolnick. Boston: Little, Brown, 1986.

Bethel, Elizabeth Rauh. *Promiseland: A Century of Life in a Negro Community.* Philadelphia: Temple University Press, 1981.

Billingsley, Andrew. *Climbing Jacob's Ladder.* New York: Simon & Schuster, 1992.

Blake, Judith. *Family Structure in Jamaica.* New York: Free Press of Glencoe, 1985.

Blake, Michael. *Comparative Youth Culture.* Boston: Routledge & Kegan Paul, 1985.

Blos, Peter. "The Child Analyst Looks at the Young Adolescent." In *Twelve to Sixteen: Early Adolescents,* edited by Jerome Kagan and Robert Coles. New York: W.W. Norton, 1972.

Bluestone, Barry, and Bennett Harrison. *The Industrialization of America.* New York: Harper & Row, 1982.

Boyd, William Lowes. "What Makes Ghetto Schools Work or Not Work?" Paper presented at the conference "The Truly Disadvantaged," sponsored by the Social Science Research Council Committee for Research on the Urban Underclass and the Center for Urban Affairs and Policy Research, Northwestern University, Evanston, Ill., 19–21 October 1989, revised February 1990.

Briere, John. "The Longterm Clinical Correlates of Childhood Sexual Victimization." Paper presented at the New York Academy of Science conference, New York, January 1987.

Brittany, A., and Mary Maynard. *Sexism, Racism and Oppression.* New York: Basil Blackwell, 1984.

Brooks-Gunn, J., and E. Reiter. "The Role of Pubertal Processes in the Early Adolescent Transition." In *The Developing Adolescent,* edited by S. Feldman and G. Elliott. Cambridge, Mass.: Harvard University Press, 1990.

Brown, Claude. "Return to Mean Streets." *Los Angeles Times,* 30 June 1986, 1B–2B.

Burton, Linda M., and Vern L. Bengston. "Black Grandmothers: Issues of Timing and Continuity of Roles." In *Grandparenthood,* edited by Vern L. Bengston and J. Robertson. Newbury Park, Calif.: Sage Publications, 1985.

Card, Josefina J., and Lauress L. Wise. "Teenage Mothers and Teenage Fathers: The Impact of Early Childbearing on the Parents' Personal and Professional Lives." In *Teenage Sexuality, Pregnancy, and Childbearing,* edited by Frank F. Furstenberg Jr., Richard Lincoln, and Jane Menken. Philadelphia: University of Pennsylvania Press, 1981.

Caughey, James L. *Imaginary Social Worlds.* Lincoln: University of Nebraska Press, 1984.

Cazanave, Noel. "Men in America: The Quest for Manhood." In *Black Families,* 1st ed., edited by Harriet Pipes McAdoo. Newbury Park, Calif.: Sage Publications, 1981.

Children's Defense Fund. *The Problems of Teenage Pregnancy, National Overview.* Washington, D.C.: Children's Defense Fund, 1988.

Chilman, C. *Adolescent Sexuality in a Changing Society,* 2d ed. New York: Wiley, 1983.

Chodorow, Nancy. *The Reproduction of Mothering.* Berkeley: University of California Press, 1978.

Clark, M. L. "Friendships and Peer Relations of Black Adolescents." In *Black Adolescents*, edited by Reginald L. Jones. Berkeley: University of California Press, 1989.

Cole, Johnetta B. "Commonalities and Differences." In *All American Women: Lines That Divide, Ties That Bind*, edited by Johnetta B. Cole. New York: Free Press, 1986.

Coles, Robert, and Geoffrey Stokes. *Sex and the American Teenager.* New York: Harper & Row, 1985.

Collins, Patricia Hill. "The Meaning of Motherhood in Black Culture and Black Mother/Daughter Relationships." *Sage* 5, no. 2 (fall 1987): 3–10.

———. *Black Feminist Thought.* New York: Routledge, 1991.

Connell, R. W. *Gender and Power: Society, the Person, and Sexual Politics.* Stanford: Stanford University Press, 1987.

Cortes, Ron. "The $10 Million Teenage Director." *Philadelphia Inquirer,* 3 July 1990, 20–21.

Costello, Cynthia, and Anne J. Stone, eds. *The American Woman, 1994–95.* New York: W.W. Norton, 1994.

Crouchett, Lawrence P., Lonnie G. Bunch III, and Martin Kendall Winnacker. *The History of the East Bay Afro-American Community, 1852–1977.* Oakland: Northern California Center for Afro-American History and Life, 1989.

Cutwright, Phillips. "Illegitimacy and Income Supplements." In *Studies in Public Welfare*, paper 12, pt. I, 90, Joint Economic Committee of the Congress, edited by R. Lerman and A. Townsend. Washington, D.C.: U.S. Government Printing Office, 1973.

Cvetknovitch, G., and B. Grote. "Psychological Development and the Social Problem of Teenage Illegitimacy." In *Adolescent Pregnancy and Childbearing: Findings from Research*, edited by C. Chilman. Washington, D.C.: U.S. Department of Health and Human Services, 1980.

Dash, Leon. "Black Teenage Pregnancy in Washington, D.C." *International Social Science Review* 61 (autumn 1986): 4.

Davidson, Laurie, and Laura Kramer Gordon. *The Sociology of Gender.* Chicago: Rand McNally College Publishing, 1979.

Davis, Patricia, and Robert O'Harrow Jr. "The Hard Path from Welfare." *The Washington Post,* 17 February 1994, 7–8.

Dawson, Deborah Anne. "The Effects of Sex Education on Adolescent Behavior." *Family Planning Perspectives* 18, no. 4 (July–August 1986): 45–50.

Degler, Carl N. *At Odds: Women and the Family in America from the Revolution to the Present.* New York: Oxford University Press, 1980.

Dent, David J. "The New Black Suburbs." *New York Times Magazine,* 14 June 1992, 22.

Denzin, Norman. "On the Ethics of Disguised Observation." *Social Problems* 15 (1968): 502–504.

De Witt, Karen. "Wave of Suburban Growth Is Being Fed by Minorities." *New York Times,* 15 August 1994, A1, A12.

Diamond, Irene, ed. *Introduction to Families, Politics, and Public Policy.* New York: Longman, 1983.

Duncan, G. J., and Willard Rodgers. "Single-Parent Families: Are Their Economic Problems Transitory or Persistent?" *Family Planning Perspectives* 19, no. 4 (July–August 1987): 50–55.

Duster, Troy. "Diversity and Multiculturalism in Higher Education: Can We Elevate the Dialog and Address the Experience?" Speech presented at University of Southern California, 30 November 1992.

Elise, Sharon. "Teenage Mothers: A Sense of Self." In *African American Single Mothers: Understanding Their Lives and Families,* edited by Bette J. Dickerson. Newbury Park, Calif.: Sage Publications, 1995.

Ellwood, David T. *Poor Support: Poverty in the American Family.* New York: Basic Books, 1988.

Ellwood, David T, and Lawrence H. Summers. "Poverty in America: Is Welfare the Answer or the Problem?" In *Fighting Poverty: What Works and What Doesn't,* edited by Sheldon H. Danzinger and Daniel H. Weinberg. Cambridge, Mass: Harvard University Press, 1986.

Evans, Sara. *Personal Politics.* New York: Vintage Books, 1979.

Fine, Michele. "Silencing in Public Schools." *Language Arts* 64 (1987): 157–174.

———. "Sexuality, Schooling, and Adolescent Females: The Missing Discourse of Desire." *Harvard Educational Review* 58, no. 1 (February 1988): 64.

Fischer, Lucy Rose. *Linked Lives: Adult Daughters and Their Mothers.* New York: Harper & Row, 1987.

Folbre, Nancy. "The Pauperization of Motherhood: Patriarchy and Public Policy in the United States." *Review of Radical Political Economics* 16, no. 4 (winter 1984): 12.

Fox, Greer Litton, and Judith K. Inazu. "Patterns and Outcomes of Mother-Daughter Communication about Sexuality." *Journal of Social Issues* 36, no. 1 (1980): 113.

Franklin, John Hope. "A Historical Note on Black Families." In *Black Families,* 2d ed., edited by Harriet Pipes McAdoo. Newbury Park, Calif.: Sage Publications, 1988.

Franklin, Raymond S. *Shadows of Race and Class.* Minneapolis: University of Minnesota Press, 1991.

Freedman, Alix M. "Habit Forming, Fast-food Chains Play a Central Role in Diet of the Inner-City Poor." *New York Times,* 19 December 1990, 1, 4.

Fuchs, Victor. *How We Live: Economic Perspectives on Americans from Birth to Death*. Cambridge, Mass.: Harvard University Press, 1983.

Furstenberg, Frank, Jr. "Burdens and Benefits: Impact of Early Childbearing on the Family." *Journal of Social Issues* 36 no. 1 (1980): 123–135.

Furstenberg, Frank, Jr., and Albert G. Crawford. "Family Support: Helping Teenage Mothers to Cope." In *Teenage Sexuality*, edited by Frank Furstenberg Jr., Richard Lincoln, and Jane Menken. Philadelphia: University of Pennsylvania Press, 1981.

Galavotti, Christine. "Predictors of Risk-Taking, Preventive Behavior and Contraceptive Use among Inner-City Adolescents." Ph.D. diss., University of California, Berkeley, 1987.

Garfinkel, Irwin, and Sara S. McLanahan. *Single Mothers and Their Children: A New American Dilemma*. Washington D.C.: The Urban Institute, 1986.

Gary, Lawrence E. "A Social Profile." In *Black Men*, edited by Lawrence E. Gary. Newbury Park, Calif.: Harper & Row, 1982.

Gibbs, Jewelle Taylor. "Conclusions and Recommendations." In *Young, Black, and Male in America*, edited by Jewelle Taylor Gibbs. Dover, Mass.: Auburn House, 1988.

Gilder, George. *Wealth and Poverty*. New York: Basic Books, 1983.

Gilligan, Carol. *In a Different Voice*. Cambridge, Mass.: Harvard University Press, 1987.

Gilligan, Carol, Nona P. Lyons, and Trudy J. Hanmer, eds. *Making Connections: The Relational Worlds of Adolescent Girls at Emma Willard School*. Cambridge, Mass.: Harvard University Press, 1990.

Glasgow, Douglas. *The Underclass: Poverty, Unemployment, and Entrapment of Ghetto Youth*. San Francisco: Jossey-Bass, 1980.

Goffman, Erving. *Stigma*. Englewood Cliffs, N.J.: Prentice Hall, 1963.

———. *Frame Analysis*. New York: Harper & Row, 1974.

Gouldner, Alvin. "Personal Reality and the Tragic Dimension in Science." In *The Sociology of Research*, edited by G. Boalth. Carbondale: Southern Illinois University Press, 1969.

Gutman, Herbert G. *The Black Family in Slavery and Freedom, 1750–1925*. New York: Random House, 1976.

Guttentag, Marcia, and Paul F. Secord. *Too Many Women? The Sex Ratio Question*. Newbury Park, Calif.: Sage Publications, 1983.

Hale-Benson, Janice. "The School Learning Environment and Academic Success." In *Black Students*, edited by Gorden LaVern Berry and Joy Keiko Asamen. Newbury Park, Calif.: Sage Publications, 1989.

Hammer, Signe. *Mothers and Daughters/Daughters and Mothers*. New York: Quadrangle, 1975.

Hanson, Shirley M. H., and Michael J. Sporokowski. "Single Parent Families." *Journal of Family Relations* 11 (January 1988): 3–8.

Hare, Nathan, and Julia Hare. *The Endangered Black Family*. San Francisco: Black Think Tank, 1984.

Harrington, Michael. *The New American Poverty*. New York: Penguin Books, 1986.

Hartley, Shirley Foster. *Illegitimacy*. Berkeley: University of California Press, 1983.

Herek, Gregory M. "On Heterosexual Masculinity: Some Psychical Consequences of the Social Construction of Gender and Sexuality." In *Changing Men,* edited by Michael S. Kimmel. Newbury Park, Calif.: Sage Publications, 1987.

Herzog, James M. "Boys Who Make Babies." In *Adolescent Parenthood,* edited by Max Sugar. New York: Spectrum Publications, 1984.

Hochschild, Arlie Russell. "The Sociology of Feeling and Emotions: Selected Possibilities." In *Another Voice,* edited by Marcia Millman. New York: Anchor Books, 1975.

Hofferth, S. L., J. R. Kahn, and W. Baldwin. "Premarital Sexual Activity among Teenage Women over the Past Three Decades." *Family Planning Perspectives* 19 (1988): 46.

Hogan, Dennis P., and Evelyn M. Kitagawa. "The Impact of Social Status, Family Structure, and Neighborhood on the Fertility of Black Adolescents." *American Journal of Sociology* 90 (1985): 831.

hooks, bell. *Ain't I a Woman?* Boston: South End Press, 1981.

Horowitz, Ruth. *Teen Mothers: Citizens or Dependents*. Chicago: University of Chicago Press, 1995.

Humphreys, Laud. *Tearoom Trade: Impersonal Sex in Public Places*, 2d ed. Chicago: Aldine, 1975.

Ianni, Francis A. J. *The Search for Structure: A Report on American Youth Today*. New York: Free Press, 1989.

Irvine, Jacqueline Jordan. *Black Students and School Failure: Policies, Practices, and Prescription*. New York: Greenwood Press, 1990.

Janowitz, Morris. *Social Control of the Welfare State*. Chicago: University of Chicago Press, 1976.

Jaynes, Gerald David, and Robin M. Williams. *A Common Destiny: Blacks and American Society*. Washington, D.C.: National Academy, 1989.

Johnson, Sylvia T. "Extra-School Factors in Achievement, Attainment, and Aspirations among Junior and Senior High School School-Aged Black Youth." Paper prepared for the Committee on the Status of Black Americans, National Research Council, Washington, D.C., 1987.

Jones, Elise F. *Teenage Pregnancy in Industrial Countries*. New Haven, Conn.: Yale University Press, 1986.

Joseph, Gloria L. "Mothers and Daughters: Traditional and New Perspectives." *Sage* 1 no. 2 (fall 1984): 17–21.

Kaplan, Elaine Bell. "Where Does a 15-year-old Mother Turn?" *Feminist Issues* 8, no. 1 (spring 1988): 51–83.

———. "Women's Perceptions of the Adolescent Experience." *Adolescence* (in press).

Kessler, R.C., and P.D. Cleary. "Social Class and Psychological Distress." *American Sociological Review* 45 (1980): 463–477.

Kisker, Ellen Eliason. "Teenagers Talk about Sex, Pregnancy and Contraception." *Family Planning Perspectives* 17, no. 2 (March–April 1985): 89.

Kotlowitz, Alex. *There Are No Children Here: The Story of Two Boys Growing Up in the Other America.* New York: Anchor Books, 1991.

Kozol, Jonathan. *Savage Inequalities: Children in America's Schools.* New York: Crown, 1991.

Ladner, Joyce, and Ruby Morton Gourdine. "Intergenerational Teenage Motherhood: Some Preliminary Findings." *Sage,* fall 1984, 22–24.

Lasch, Christopher. *Haven in a Heartless Land.* New York: Basic Books, 1972.

Leonard, Linda. *The Wounded Woman.* Athens: Ohio University Press, Swallow Press, 1982.

Levitan, Lar A. *Program in Aid of the Poor,* 8th ed. Baltimore: Johns Hopkins Press, 1981.

Lewis Lapham. *Money and Class in America.* New York: Ballantine Books, 1988.

Lewis, Oscar. "The Culture of Poverty." *Scientific American* 215 (October 1966): 19–25.

Liebow, Elliot. *Tally's Corner.* Boston: Little, Brown, 1975.

Lindermann, W. J., and L. Scott. "Wanted and Unwanted Pregnancy in Early Adolescence: Evidence from a Clinic Population." *Journal of Early Adolescence* 1 (1983).

Lips, Hilary M. *Women, Men and Power.* London: Mayfield Publishing, 1991.

Luker, Kristen. *Taking Chances: Abortion and the Decision Not to Contracept.* Berkeley: University of California Press, 1975.

———. "Understanding the Risk-Taker." *The Family Planner* 30 (summer 1977): 1–2.

———. *Deceptive Conceptions.* Cambridge, Mass.: Harvard University Press, 1996.

MacLeod, Jay. *Ain't No Makin' It: Leveled Aspirations in a Low-Income Neighborhood.* Boulder: Westview Press, 1987.

McGrory, Mary. "What to Do about Parents of Illegitimate Children." *The Washington Post,* 15 February 1994, 25.

McLanahan, Sara. "Family Structure and Stress: A Longitudinal Comparison of Two-Parent and Female-Headed Families." *Journal of Marriage and the Family* 9 (1983): 25.

Mead, Lawrence M. *Beyond Entitlement: The Social Obligations of Citizenship.* New York: Free Press, 1986.

Merida, Kevin, and Kenneth J. Cooper. "Black Lawmakers Sound the Alarm." *Washington Post,* February 1994, 9.

Michelson, Roslyn A., and Stephen Samuel Smith. "Inner-City Social Dislocation and School Outcomes: A Structural Interpretation." In *Black Students,* edited by Gordon LaVern Berry and Joy Keiko Asamen. Newbury Park, Calif.: Sage Publications, 1989.

Miller, Warren B. "Psychological Vulnerability to Unwanted Pregnancy." In *Teenage Sexuality,* edited by Frank Furstenberg Jr., Richard Lincoln, and Jane Menken. Philadelphia: University of Pennsylvania Press, 1981.

Mills, C. Wright. *The Sociological Imagination.* New York: Oxford University Press, 1959.

Moore, Kristin A. "The Effect of Government Policies on Out-of-Wedlock Sex and Pregnancy." *Family Planning Perspectives* 9 (1977): 16.

Moore, Kristin A., and Martha R. Burt. *Private Crisis, Public Cost: Policy Perspectives on Teenage Childbearing.* Washington, D.C.: Urban Institute, 1982.

Moore, Kristin A., Angela Romano, and Cheryl Oakes. *Child Trends, Inc.* Washington, D.C.: National Center for Health Statistics, Department of Health and Human Services, 1994.

Morgan, David L. "Strategies and Sociologists: A Comment on Crow." *Sociology* 23 (1989): 25–29.

Morgan, Phyliss Evelyn. "The Church of God Minister's Perception of Unwed, Teenage Pregnancy in the Church and Community." Ph.D. diss., University of California, Berkeley, 1985.

Moynihan, Daniel P. *The Negro Family: The Case for National Action.* Washington, D.C.: U.S. Government Printing Office, 1965.

———. *Family and Nation: The Godkin Lectures at Harvard University.* San Diego: Harcourt Brace Jovanovich, 1987.

Murray, Charles. *Losing Ground: American Social Policy, 1950–1980.* New York: Basic Books, 1984.

Musick, Judith S. "The High-Stakes Challenge of Programs for Adolescent Mothers." In *Adolescence and Poverty: Challenges of the 1990s,* edited by Peter Edelman and Joyce Ladner. Washington, D.C.: Center for National Policy Press, 1991.

———. *Young, Poor, and Pregnant: The Psychology of Teenage Motherhood.* New Haven, Conn.: Yale University Press, 1993.

Oakley, Ann. "Interviewing Women: A Contradiction in Terms." In *Doing Feminist Research,* edited by Helen Roberts. Boston: Routledge & Kegan Paul, 1981.

Ogbu, John. *Minority Education and Caste.* New York: Academic Press, 1978.

Passell, Peter. "Economic Trends." *New York Times,* 20 June 1996, 2.

Pearce, Diane. "The Feminization of Ghetto Poverty." *Society* 5 (November–December 1983): 24–27.

"Percentage Comparison of African American and White Families Affected by Unemployment, 1988." *The State of Black America, 1990,* January 1990, p. 218.

Philliber, Susan Gustavus. "Socialization for Childbearing." *Journal of Social Issue* 36, no. 1 (1980): 230–245.

Pittman, Karen. *Adolescent Pregnancy: An Anatomy of a Social Problem in Search of Comprehensive Solutions.* Washington, D.C.: Children's Defense Fund, 1987.

Pittman, Karen, and Gina Adams. *Teenage Pregnancy: An Advocate's Guide to the Numbers.* Washington, D.C.: Children's Defense Fund, 1988.

———. *What about the Boys? Teenage Pregnancy Prevention Strategies.* Washington, D. C.: Children's Defense Fund, 1988.

Piven, Frances Fox, and Richard A. Cloward. *Regulating the Poor: The Function of Public Welfare.* New York: Vintage Books, 1993.

Placek, Paul J., and Gerry E. Hendershot. "Public Welfare and Family Planning: An Empirical Study of the Brood Sow Myth." *Social Problems* 23 (1975): 226.

Rank, Mark Robert. *Living on the Edge: The Realities of Welfare in America.* New York: Columbia University Press, 1994.

Reichelt, P., and H. Werley. "Contraception, Abortion, and Venereal Disease: Teenagers' Knowledge and the Effect of Education." *Family Planning Perspectives* 7 (1975): 83–88.

Reid, John. "Blacks in America in the 1980s." *Population Bulletin* 37 (December 1982): 27.

Reinhartz, Shulamit. *On Becoming a Social Scientist: From Survey Research and Participant Observation to Experiential Analysis.* San Francisco: Jossey–Bass, 1979.

Richel, A.V. *Teen Pregnancy and Parenting.* New York: Hemisphere Publishing, 1989.

Ries, Paula, and Anne J. Stone, eds. *The American Woman, 1992–93: A Status Report.* New York: W.W. Norton, 1992.

Robbins, James. "Black Families: Identifying the Special Strengths—and Needs—of the Black Family." *Christian Science Monitor,* 16 May 1986, 2.

Rogers, Joseph. "Fighting Back: Nine Modes of Adaptation of a Deviant Label." *Social Problems* 33, no. 3 (January–February 1982): 111–123.

Ross, H.L., and I. Sawhill. *Time of Transition: The Growth of Families Headed by Women.* Washington, D.C.: Urban Institute, 1975.

Rothenberg, Paula S. "The Prison of Race and Gender: Stereotypes, Ideology, Language, and Social Control." In *Racism and Sexism: An Integrated Study,* edited by Paula S. Rothenberg. New York: St. Martin's Press, 1988.

Ruben, Lillian. *Worlds of Pain.* New York: Basic Books, 1976.

Russo, Nancy F. "The Motherhood Mandate." *Journal of Social Issues* 32 (1976): 143–153.

Sachs, Barbara Ann. "The Relationship of Cognitive Development to Inter- personal Problem Solving Abilities in Female Adolescents." Ph.D. diss., University of California, Berkeley, 1981.

Salguero, Carlo. "The Role of Ethnic Factors in Adolescent Pregnancy and Motherhood." In *Adolescent Parenthood,* edited by Max Sugar. New York: Spectrum Publications, 1984.

Sattel, Jack W. "Men, Inexpressiveness, and Power." In *Feminist Frontiers,* edited by Laurel Richardson and Verta Taylor. New York: Random House, 1986.

Sawyer, Ethel. "Methodological Problems in Studying So-Called 'Deviant' Communities." In *The Death of White Sociology,* edited by Joyce Ladner. New York: Random House, 1973.

Schur, Edwin. *Labeling Women Deviant.* Philadelphia: Temple University Press, 1983).

Scott-Jones, Diane. "Black Families and the Education of Black Children: Current Issues." Paper commissioned by the Committee on the Status of Black Americans, National Research Council, Washington, D.C., 1987.

Senderovitz, Judith, and John M. Paxman. "Adolescent Fertility: Worldwide Concerns." *Population Bulletin* 40, no. 2 (April 1985): 22.

Sidel, Ruth. *Women and Children Last.* New York: Viking Penguin, 1986.

Simmons, Charlene. "Custodial vs. Non-Custodial Parents: A Case Study of Family Support Division, Sacramento County, California." Ph.D. diss., University of California, Berkeley, 1986.

Simmons, Robert, and Frances Rosenberg. "Disturbance in the Self-Image at Adolescence." *American Sociological Review* 38 (1973): 553–568.

Sklar, Jane, and Beth Berkow. "Teenage Family Formation in Postwar Amer- ica." *Family Planning Perspectives* 6 (1974): 80.

Smith, Althea, and Abigail J. Stewart. "Approaches to Studying Racism and Sexism in Black Women's Lives." *Journal Of Social Issues* 39, no. 3 (1983): 1–15.

Smith, E.A., and J.R. Udry. "Coital and Non-Coital Sexual Behaviors of White and Black Adolescents." *American Journal of Public Health* 32 (1986): 234–256.

Snyder, Mark. "Self-Fulfilling Stereotypes." In *Racism and Sexism: An Inte- grated Study,* edited by Paula S. Rothenberg. New York: St. Martin's Press, 1988.

Solinger, Richie. *Wake Up Little Susie: Single Pregnancy and Race before Roe v. Wade.* New York: Routledge, 1992.

Spady, William G. "The Impact of School Resources on Students." In *Review of Research in Education*, vol. 1, edited by Fred N. Kerlinger. Ithaca, Ill.: F.E. Peacock.

Stack, Carol. *All Our Kin*. New York: Harper and Row, 1974.

Staples, Robert. *Masculinity*. San Francisco: Scholar Press, 1982.

———. "Changes in Black Family Structure: The Conflict between Family Ideology and Structural Conditions." *Journal of Marriage and the Family* 47 (November 1985): 1005–1013.

Statistical Abstract of the United States, 1994, 114th ed., table 71. Washington, D. C.: Bureau of the Census.

Stewart, Pearl. "Bleak Report on Oakland's Single Mothers." *San Francisco Chronicle*, 13 May 1986, 3.

———. "Guards at Apartment Give Up Their Shotguns." *San Francisco Chronicle*, 5 September 1987, 3.

Stolberg, Sheryl. "Teen Pregnancies Force Town to Grow Up." *Los Angeles Times*, 29 November 1996, A56–A57.

Strauss, Anselm L. *Qualitative Analysis for Social Science*. New York: Cambridge University Press, 1987.

Sum, Andrew M., and W. Neal Fogg. "The Adolescent Poor and the Transition to Early Adulthood." In *Adolescence and Poverty: Challenges of the 1990s*, edited by Peter Edelman and Joyce Ladner. Washington, D.C.: Center for National Policy Press, 1991.

Taylor, Ronald L. "Black Youth In Crisis." In *The Black Family*, 5th ed., edited by Robert Staples. Belmont, Calif.: Wadworth, 1994.

Thompson, Daniel. *The Sociology of the Family*. New York: Dial Press, 1980.

Tobin, Gary A. *Divided Neighborhoods: Changing Patterns of Racial Segregation*. Newbury Park, Calif.: Sage Publications, 1987.

deTocqueville, Alexis. *Democracy in America*. Edited by J.P. Meyer. New York: Doubleday Anchor Books, 1969.

Tolson, Andrew. *The Limits of Masculinity*. New York: Harper & Row, 1977.

Troutt, David Dante. *The Thin Red Line*. San Francisco: West Coast Regional Office, Consumers Union of the U. S., 1993.

Trussell, James. "Teenage Pregnancy in the United States." In *Readings on Teenage Pregnancy from Family Planning Perspectives, 1985 through 1989*. New York: Alan Guttmacher Institute, 1990.

Tucker, M. Belinda, and Claudia Mitchell-Kernan, eds. *The Decline in Marriage among African Americans*. New York: Russell Sage Foundation, 1995.

Vinovskis, Marie A. "An 'Epidemic' of Adolescent Pregnancy? Some Historical Considerations." *Journal of Family History* 6, no. 2 (summer 1981): 205–230.

Wallace, Michele. *Black Macho and the Myth of the Super Woman*. New York: Dial Press, 1978.

Welbourne, A. F.. "The Relation of Parental Sexual Knowledge and Attitudes and Communication about Sexual Topics with their Early Adolescent Children." Ph.D. diss., New York University, 1977.

Westney, Quida E., Reness R. Jenkins, June Dobbs Butts, and Irving Williams. "Dating and Sexual Patterns, Sexual Development and Behavior in Black Preadolescents." In *Young, Black and Male in America: An Endangered Species,* edited by Reginald Jones. Dover, Mass.: Auburn House, 1988.

Whelehan, Imelda. *Modern Feminist Thought: From The Second Wave to Post-Feminism.* New York: New York University Press, 1995.

Whitman, David. "Liberal Rhetoric and the Welfare Underclass." *Society* 24 (November–December 1983): 12.

Williams, Terry, and William Kornblum. *Growing Up Poor.* Lexington, Mass.: Lexington Books, 1985.

Wilson, William J. *The Truly Disadvantaged.* Chicago: University of Chicago Press, 1987.

Zill, Nicholas, and Christine Winquist Nord. *Running in Place: How American Families Are Faring in a Changing Economy and an Individualistic Society.* Washington, D.C.: Child Trends, Inc., 1994.

Index

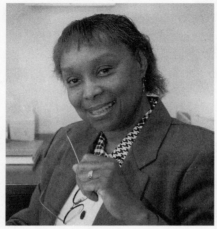

Elaine Bell Kaplan

Elaine Bell Kaplan received her bachelor's degree in sociology/psychology at Baruch College, CUNY, and her master's and Ph.D. degrees from the University of California at Berkeley. She is an assistant professor of sociology at the University of Southern California. She has written articles on gender, race, and class issues as they are experienced by women of color, Black domestic workers, Black working-class mothers and their families, and Black single mothers, and on Black, Latina, and White women's perceptions of their adolescent experiences. She is presently engaged in researching and writing on how Black, Latina, and White girls experience their adolescent development. She lives in Los Angeles with her husband and her son.

Compositor: Publication Services, Inc.
Text: 11/13.5 Caledonia
Display: Caledonia
Printer: Maple-Vail Book Manufacturing Group
Binder: Maple-Vail Book Manufacturing Group